SO-BAY-216

Previous praise for Sonya Huber's
Cover Me: A Health Insurance Memoir

"*Cover Me* is the best kind of memoir; it is engaging, enraging,
tragic, and funny. Fortunately, laughter as medicine is one thing
the insurance companies have not yet managed to deny."
—T. Tamara Weinstein, *Elevate Difference*

"Wise, irreverent, honest, and utterly compelling. . . . Sonya Huber
finds unexpected truth and gentle comedy in every bizarre corner
of this insane labyrinth we call our health-care system."
—Dinty W. Moore, author of *Between Panic and Desire*

"What I found so compelling about Huber's story is her ability to make
the personal resonate so much more loudly than the political ideas or
theories, while capably insuring that her own story underscores her
political stance on health care. I found myself wanting to send
copies to every member of the House and Senate."
—Sarah Werthan, *Brevity Book Reviews*

"The sheer, jet-propelled energy of this memoir elevates it into
a tour de force. I found it by turns hilarious and heartbreaking."
—Sue William Silverman, author of
Fearless Confessions: A Writer's Guide to Memoir

"Huber's sure-footed prose considers how deeply connected an
individual's health is to being both rooted and free, confident or
fearful of securing even the most routine treatment. Once covered,
she is safe under that blanket of care, and wise enough to
understand that covers are easily blown, or blown away."
—Lisa Romeo, *ForeWord Reviews*

"Huber's irreverent humor makes her provocative
'health insurance memoir' worth a read."
—Karen Springen, *Booklist*

"This book illustrates, in a way that mere political rhetoric cannot, how the lack of accessible, affordable medical care negatively affects everyone on a personal, emotional, and economic scale."
—Joan Hanna, *Author Exposure*

"Timely, passionate, informative, and moving, Sonya Huber's *Cover Me* is a scathing memoir of an uninsured young mother's encounter with health care in America."
—Floyd Skloot, author of *In the Shadow of Memory*

"In this humorous and affecting memoir, Huber details her experiences navigating the American health care system and brings a necessary dose of reality to the political debates and propaganda surrounding health care reform."
—Women and Children First Bookstore

PAIN WOMAN
TAKES YOUR KEYS
AND OTHER ESSAYS FROM
A NERVOUS SYSTEM

AMERICAN LIVES
Series editor: Tobias Wolff

PAIN WOMAN

TAKES YOUR KEYS

AND OTHER ESSAYS FROM

A NERVOUS SYSTEM

Sonya Huber

University of Nebraska Press | Lincoln & London

© 2017 by the Board of Regents of the
University of Nebraska

Acknowledgments for the use of copyrighted
material appear on page xi, which constitutes
an extension of the copyright page.

All rights reserved
Manufactured in the United States of America

Library of Congress Cataloging-in-Publication Data
Names: Huber, Sonya, 1971– author.
Title: Pain woman takes your keys, and other
essays from a nervous system / Sonya Huber.
Description: Lincoln: University of Nebraska
Press, 2017. | Series: American lives |
Includes bibliographical references.
Identifiers: LCCN 2016034811 (print)
LCCN 2016055108 (ebook)
ISBN 9780803299917 (paperback: alk. paper)
ISBN 9781496200839 (epub)
ISBN 9781496200846 (mobi)
ISBN 9781496200853 (pdf)
Subjects: LCSH: Chronic pain. | BISAC:
LITERARY COLLECTIONS / Essays. |
HEALTH & FITNESS / Physical Impairments.
Classification: LCC PS3608.U246 P35 2017 (print) |
LCC PS3608.U246 (ebook) | DDC 814/.6—dc23
LC record available at https://lccn.loc.gov/2016034811

Designed and set in
Garamond Premier Pro by L. Auten.

Pain is important: how we evade it, how we succumb to it, how we deal with it, how we transcend it.

—Audre Lorde, *Conversations with Audre Lorde*

CONTENTS

Preface   ix

Acknowledgments   xi

I. Pain Bows in Greeting

What Pain Wants   3

The Lava Lamp of Pain   7

Welcome to the Kingdom of the Sick   18

The Alphabet of Pain   21

Prayer to Pain   36

II. Side Projects and Secret Identities

My Alternate Selves with Pain in
Silver Lamé Bodysuits   41

The Cough Drop and the
Puzzle of Modernity   44

From Inside the Egg   50

Cupcakes   60

Amoeba Girl   66

III. **My Machines**

The Status of Pain   71

Peering into the Dark of the Self,
with Selfie   79

Augmentation   87

Interstate and Interbeing   98

Pain Woman Takes Your Keys   100

IV. **Bitchiness as Treatment Protocol**

On Gratitude, and Off   107

Life Is Good[1,2,3]   115

Dear Noted Feminist Scholar   117

V. **Intimate Moments with the Three of Us**

A Pain-Sex Anti-Manifesto   121

The Joy of Not Cooking   129

Kidney Stone in My Shoe   134

If Woman Is Five   138

A Day in the Grammar of Disease   146

VI. **Measuring the Sky**

Vital Sign 5   151

Alternative Pain Scale   155

In the Grip of the Sky   158

Between One and Ten Thousand   160

Inside the Nautilus   171

Sources   179

PREFACE

This is a collection of unconventional essays on chronic pain; my goal with these essays was not to fix or provide advice (most of us have had too much of that) but to explore the landscape. Pain is a territory known by those who are in that land. I am in a small corner of it, and the more I see of its vastness, the more I realize how little I know. I hope that in trying to put my own experience into words, I am not confounding or isolating anyone else in pain. I hope with these essays to add to the growing literature about what pain is and how it is experienced, imagined, and expressed so that its universal burden can be shared. Above all, I hope to connect with other people who have visited the land of pain or who are there now, to help us collectively understand this experience that is an inextricable part of being human, and to build treatment models for addressing pain that are humane and comprehensive as our scientific and emotional understanding of pain grows. And I hope this book is not depressing; I had so much fun writing it.

Nalini Jones, Elizabeth Hilts, Rachel Basch, and Sandy Rodriguez Barron have delved deeply into this topic with me, offering insights and encouragement at every step; my dear friend Elizabeth, in particular, walks and texts the journey with me, every painful step, and I love her more than words can say. Martha Bayne and Zoe Zolbrod at the *Rumpus* were generous enough to consider a second version of "The Lava Lamp of Pain" after the first one didn't work, and that publication and the response from it gave me the impetus to follow all the metaphors. Thanks to Dinty W. Moore at *Brevity*, Joe Mackall at *River Teeth*, Jennifer Niesslein at *Full Grown People*, Hattie Fletcher at *Creative Nonfiction*, and Michael Steinberg for their continued encouragement and support, and all the other editors who allowed me to connect with readers, which has been more important with this collection than anything else I've written. Thank you in particular to Alicia Christensen, Rosemary Vestal, Joeth Zucco, and everyone else at University of Nebraska Press, as well as fantastic copy editor Patty Beutler. Thank you to Dennis Keenan for sharing Elaine Scarry's work with me. I wanted to offer specific and huge thanks to readers who have been in pain who took the time to comment on an essay or a blog post or send me an email; your words are the reason I kept going with what seemed at first like an impossible project. You each helped me understand that I was expressing something true. Thanks to Stan, Heidi, Glenn, Nicole, Meg, and Rosarita Huber, and to Jon and Terry Price for their support, as well as to my colleagues at Fairfield University, and my friends near and far, including Jocelyn, Anna, Gwen, Emily, Kris, and Bryan. A special thanks to everyone who gave me stickers for my cane. Thank you to the patient advocates, including Kelly of RA Warrior and the moderators of online forums, and to researchers and doctors who advocate for comprehensive pain care. Thank you to Dr. Rose, Dr. Strohmayer, Dr. Rzucidlo, Dr. Lyddy, and Dr. Snowden for their excellent, responsive, and respectful medical care; good doctors who see their patients as people and listen are true artists. Thank you to my Buddhist teacher Dzigar Kongtrul Rinpoche, Elizabeth Mattis Nyamgal, and the Mangala Shri Bhuti sangha. Thank you to fellow disability writers everywhere, in particular Sarah Einstein and Karrie Higgins for their inspiration, and Andrea Scarpino for her beautiful poetry. My biggest thanks to Cliff Price and Ivan for their understanding and for helping me carry the pain and laughing with me through it.

ACKNOWLEDGMENTS

"What Pain Wants" appeared in *Rogue Agent Journal*

"The Lava Lamp of Pain" appeared in *The Rumpus*

"Prayer to Pain" is forthcoming in *Passages North*

"Amoeba Girl" appeared in *Eleven Eleven*

"The Status of Pain" appeared in *Full Grown People*

"Pain Woman Takes Your Keys" appeared on Michael Steinberg's blog

"Life Is Good[1,2,3]" appeared in *DIAGRAM*

"The Joy of Not Cooking" appeared in *Role Reboot*

"Kidney Stone in My Shoe" appeared in *VIDA*

"If Woman Is Five" appeared in *River Teeth*

"A Day in the Grammar of Disease" appeared in *Brevity*

"In the Grip of the Sky" appeared in *Creative Nonfiction*

PAIN WOMAN
TAKES YOUR KEYS
AND OTHER ESSAYS FROM
A NERVOUS SYSTEM

I

PAIN BOWS IN GREETING

WHAT PAIN WANTS

Pain wants you to put in earplugs because sounds are grating.

Pain has something urgent to tell you but forgets over and over again what it was.

Pain tells you to put your laptop in the refrigerator.

Pain runs into walls at forty-five-degree angles and ricochets back into the center of the room.

Pain resents being personified or anthropomorphized.

Pain is a four-dimensional person with fractal intelligence.

Pain wants to be taken to an arts and crafts store.

Pain likes to start big projects and not finish them.

Pain wants to clean one countertop.

Pain asks you to break itself up into neat, square segments like a chocolate bar.

Pain makes a hissing, popping hum like high-tension power lines.

Pain has ambition but is utterly unfocused.

Pain will get its revenge if you ignore it but sometimes forgets what it was angry about.

Pain wants to watch a different channel than you do on TV.

Pain looks at you with the inscrutable eyes and thin beak of an egret.

Pain stubs out the cigarette of your to-do list.

Pain will first try to do some things on that list but will end up
   with socks on its antlers.

Pain demands that you make eye contact with it and then
   sit utterly still.

Pain folds the minutes into fascinating origami constructions
   with its long fingers.

Pain leaves the meter running.

Pain asks you to think about the breath flowing in and
   out of your lungs.

Pain will ask you to do this 307 times today.

Pain does not mean any harm to you.

Pain is frustrated that it is trapped in a body that is ill-fitting
   for its unfolded shape.

Pain has been born in the wrong universe.

Pain is wild with grief at the discomfort it causes.

Pain wants to collect bottle caps to show you the serrated edges,
   which mean something it cannot explain.

Pain keeps pointing to serrated edges and scalloped patterns
   but cannot explain how these will unlock it.

Pain emphasizes that it is not a god, but then makes the symbol for
   "neighbor" over and over, and you do not understand
   what it means.

Pain puts its beaked head in its long-fingered wing hands in
frustration and loneliness.

Pain winks at you with its dot-black eyes and tries to make the
sign for "I love you."

Pain folds up its wings and legs and spindles quietly and blinks
up at you when you say, "I know."

Pain understands that you cannot say "I love you" back but that
there is something bigger behind "I love you" that you do not
have the words for.

Pain also understands that the background to "I love you"
is something like a highway.

Pain licks at its hot spots like an anxious dog.

Pain, when held in place, spirals down into drill bits,
so it has to keep moving to prevent these punctures.

Pain asks you to breathe deeply so it can zing about and not get
caught on the edges and corners of calendars, books,
and electronic rectangles.

Pain's favorite music is the steel drum, and its favorite flavor is fig.

Pain prefers any texture in which tiny seeds are embedded.

Pain shakes its head—no, it says, that is *you* who likes that texture—
and will have nothing to do with spheres.

Pain wants only for you to see where it starts and you stop,
but you are a transparent bubble.

Pain and its kind have waited patiently for humans to evolve into the
fourth dimension, but they are worried the project is failing.

Pain feels as though Earth's gravity is as strong as Jupiter's.

Pain has something metallic in its bones and is captured
  by the magnetic core of our hot planet.

Pain envies flesh and its soft strength and ease of movement.

Pain inhabits curved, soft bodies in hopes of fluid movement
  and then cries when it breaks them.

Pain would like french fries and Netflix.

THE LAVA LAMP OF PAIN

Pain moved into my body five years ago. It wasn't the whack of an anvil or the burn of a scraped knee. This pain sat warmly on the surface of my hands up to the elbows like evil, pink evening gloves, with a sort of swimming cap clenched on my head, with blue plastic flowers at the base of the neck, and a nauseating blur in the eyes. At other times the pain was a cold ache at the knuckles, with a frazzle in the stomach and a steady and oblong ache from hip to hip across the pelvis. It was a rigid, curled ache in the toes like the talons of a predatory bird.

How long had it been there? I had noticed, driving home from my teaching job at a public university in a small Georgia town, that my hands hurt when I gripped the steering wheel. I decided to try to grip things more lightly.

But the achiness spread.

Maybe it was stress, I reasoned. Life had exploded in the past few years: a divorce, then single motherhood, and a mysterious infection that turned out to be Hashimoto's Thyroiditis, an autoimmune condition where the thyroid slowly erodes. As the wreckage began to settle, I seemed to be left with a glowing skeleton. I got up in the morning on a fall day, swung my legs out of bed, and thought, *Oh, the skeleton did not like that.*

Lying in bed at night, I felt my skeleton pulsing. I shifted under the sheet and struggled to fold together my collection of bones. I was a silverware drawer in a mess, a tangled wind chime. I wedged extra pillows between my knees. Advil barely helped at all. It was stress. It was tension. I took a yoga class. I was getting old.

But nobody gets old within three months. I was so angry at every limb, the way each joint refused to do my bidding.

I didn't know then that I had become a lava lamp of curling, invisible storm clouds, filled with a surge of mute motion that might be its own kind of fierce beauty.

I waited a few months and took more Advil. Maybe it was a bad flu or work stress. I still remember the moment, sitting in my car, when I realized things were seriously wrong. The pain broke through whatever container I had built for it. It was bigger. I remember taking out my cell phone and calling the doctor, saying I needed to talk to her about something. It was overcast.

I drove to her office near the Chinese-Mexican buffet. She drew vials of blood and saw that there were weird things on my blood test. She sent me two blocks down the road to a nurse practitioner near the Big Lots, who prodded my joints and explained to me that my body was engaged in a new form of self-sabotage.

I knew self-sabotage, but apparently this wasn't about apologizing too much, or dating wily, unreliable men, or trying to be perfect. This was actual physical erosion. I now had two autoimmune diseases. I was devouring myself.

The joint pain came from rheumatoid disease; my immune system saw my joints as the enemy, for reasons no one really understands.

She left after the physical exam so I could put on my clothes. I thought of my mother's aching, curling, swollen fingers and bouts of pain. I remembered my aunt's crumpled, twisted frame. I could have those bodies in the future, but the deformity threatening me in the future scared me less than the pain itself, this hooded cape that had descended, heavy like wet wool.

I was thirty-eight. I had a five-year-old son who liked to take a running start and catapult himself onto me, all soft limbs and flying hair and giggles, and nestle in and climb and wrestle.

Instead of reaching out to embrace him, I found myself stiffening against contact and wincing. "No, don't hurt Mommy."

I was the bitchy patient, crying after each doctor's appointment, crying with fear when they told me they didn't know what next. I was desperate to be the mommy I'd been before. I wanted to claw my way back to the body I knew.

Instead, I was a slave to the sky. I noticed that an impending storm could knock me flat. The barometric pressure shifts and the Georgia humidity echoed a pressure inside me. I could feel the swelling in each pocket of synovial fluid. I couldn't think or will myself through it.

On one stormy day I dropped off my son at day care and called in sick. I canceled conversations and meetings with my students.

Lying in bed, a day destroyed, I couldn't even do sickness the way I had enjoyed in the past. I couldn't read. The words swam in front of my eyes. I downloaded podcasts and flipped through them listlessly. The only ones that helped were on Buddhism and the illusion of concrete experience.

What you think is bad might not be bad. When you reject something, that rejection causes more pain than the negative experience itself.

I was so whacked out with pain that everyday objects seemed to shine. Every moment I was grateful I was still breathing. I was grateful that I could fall asleep. I was grateful when the rain broke over my rental house, and in the cool air I could get up and move a little easier.

Pain is a cloud, a mist. Pain is like the weather itself. Though the wind and the fronts are invisible, it can flatten a landscape.

The nurse practitioner put me on a drug that once was used for chemo, strong enough to suppress my immune system. I wanted that. I wanted to do battle with myself. But the pain continued.

For the pain, she gave me strong anti-inflammatories and steroids. I swallowed them gratefully at the kitchen counter each morning as I packed a lunch for my son. I felt the pain ebb, and I thought, *Take that.* I stood up straighter and felt my skeleton quiet.

After a few months the strong, white pills had messed with my liver and my guts. Lumps showed up in my inflamed liver, and red numbers showed up on worrisome blood tests. I'm told the damage will not be permanent, but the disease itself has the potential to attack my organs, my tendons, and my other vital systems.

I met a new friend named Tramadol, an opioid that I always took as prescribed. I began to look forward to the times during the day when I could take my next dose. I still have a clear memory of opening up the pill case in my purse and seeing the little, pointed ovals resting there like smiles. I'd scoop them out with a finger, swallow with a glass of water, and return for a few hours to the body I remembered.

I had moments where my body could be loose. I chased my son, fell back on the couch in laughter, and I loved my quiet skeleton.

The pain pills created an illusion. That pre-sickness body was dead, but I didn't know it.

In place of that quiet physical body, I would have to adapt to a noisy one, a body with the city-buzz of pain always in the background, a chatty, zinging body echoing with the sounds of a thousand-signal radio-buzz jackhammer, snatches-of-an-infomercial, baby-crying, Vincent-Price-ghoulish-laugh violin-cymbals. This body sang with touches of a strange symphony and an alien melody I strained to understand. Audre Lorde describes pain as visiting her "bringing all of its kinfolk," and I understood hosting that various, prickly crowd: "Not that any one of them was overwhelming, but just that all in concert, or even in small repertory groups, they were excruciating."

The noise of pain, the surge of weather-pain, crept in, wearing a heavy cloak—even with the Tramadol.

I had to leave my son's chess tournament because the pain was about to make me throw up in a third-grade classroom among the piles of jackets and the chessboards. I lost days, lying in bed, trying to work, worrying about losing work, losing money, losing my ability to support myself and him.

My nurse practitioner had given me a prescription for strong drugs to slow down and dampen my immune system, but I wanted the whole disease and its pain erased. I wanted the new neutron bombs I'd seen on upbeat drug commercials, where people with rheumatoid disease cavorted in sunlit meadows. I wanted every dangerous pharmaceutical those companies had to offer.

I wanted back each day of my present life. I wanted my hours not to be soaked in this new substance, this jagged strange distracting heat.

I needed more than a nurse practitioner, so I shopped for specialists and made appointments. I drove long distances to see them. Dr. A told me I just had very flexible joints. Dr. B told me I was a young, attractive professor who "looked great," so I had nothing to worry about. He went to get a pamphlet, and I stood up and walked out, quivering with rage.

A year into my pain adventure, I had not yet learned that the word pain is contained within patience. I was livid and panicked with the losses that had accrued.

I started having problems walking. My left hip felt like it was grinding against itself. In desperation I drove to the local pharmacy and stood in front of the rack of canes in the corner near the bedpans and boxes of gauze. I lifted up a cane decorated with gaudy purple and orange passionflowers. I set its rubber tip down on the ground with dread. I didn't want to be a slow, three-legged girl with metal tubing.

I took a step and leaned my weight on the cane. Pressure eased. I could walk with a bit more balance. I leaned on the cane and walked up to the register. I paid for the cane and clomped with it out to the car. I flung it into the passenger seat and cried.

The cane made my pain suddenly real to friends, neighbors, and colleagues. Some of them stood stock-still as I approached. They stared, understanding something communicated by a length of metal tubing that all my words had failed to say.

They asked how I was doing in the grocery store parking lot or on a walkway near the English building, and I watched as their eyes squinted slightly in fear. The reptilian part of their brains hissed and said, *Danger. Back away.*

Pain is the world's most dangerous criminal, Death's sidekick. When the Grim Reaper shuffles in, what we fear most is not the shroud but the sharp scythe he carries, the "ouch" before the silence. It's hard to confess pain, because other people feel it or imagine it. Then they want to solve it. They will tell you the same solutions over and over: have you tried yoga? I had an aunt . . .

They are desperate for the answer to the unanswerable, just like me.

Dr. C was a golden opportunity: a specialist at a fancy university medical center. He would cure me, I knew it.

I got in my car in the Georgia heat and drove along four highways and across one state line. Maybe it was the distance that let me hope I was making a pilgrimage, that each mile brought me closer to relief and to recovering the body and the self I used to be. I imagined that maybe when I got there, I would nail my cane on a wall next to the crutches in a grotto with a Virgin statue weeping real tears.

I went inside a sterile, white room and recited my list of meds to the doctor. He was busy and important and had a resident with him who watched him in adoration. He cocked an eyebrow and said, "You're on a *lot* of pain pills."

He implied that I was a med-seeker, someone bluffing symptoms to get prescriptions for pain meds for fun or to feed an addiction. I stared at him open-mouthed.

In a panic, I began to play meek, because I had already learned that a doctor's story could block the way to help. Instead of too young or too attractive, I was now needy and addicted. My chest tightened, pulse racing.

My voice shook as I told him I was only following the orders of another doctor. I wanted to tell him this was the only power I had left: to follow instructions from people who were supposed to know how to fix this.

He told me there were vague indicators of the disease but no screaming diagnosis that would lead to more serious treatments. Those serious treatments, it would turn out, were also not a cure, but at the time I wanted magic and remission. To know more, he would need an MRI. I nodded, glad to accumulate evidence. A phone call, however, confirmed that my insurance wouldn't cover the test. So the specialist sent me back to my regular doctor and wished me luck.

I went outside and stood next to my car in the parking lot of the medical center in South Carolina, and I screamed and swore. I screamed with a desperation that made my throat hoarse. I made a scene and screamed again with my wet face to the sky.

I'd been in pain every day for a year, trying to make it as a single mom with a full-time job and no family in the area. I would not be fixed. I could not be healed.

I had been driven beyond the brink of fear into anger, which was easier. I was angry at the smug doctor. But anger and rage brought me back to panic.

I screamed so loud in that parking lot that they heard me inside. Someone in that building called my doctor back in my hometown and reported me as a bad patient, a crazy patient, someone who couldn't play by the rules of decorum because I was making a scene in their parking lot with my grief and my rage over this pain I couldn't handle, over the pain of my lost life.

When I went home, the nurse practitioner began to treat me as though I were insane, as if I might snap with rage at any point, as if I didn't know the difference between a parking lot and a doctor's office, as if I had broken a rule. And I had broken several. I didn't know all the rules of pain yet, the rules of doctors and power and the military decorum and submission, but I would learn.

I had nothing to do but go back to the pain, my constant companion. Unlike the doctors, the pain itself was reliable and might be learned. As I meditated or lay in bed, I watched the way it shifted and rolled along my limbs. I learned that often when the weather report was wrong, I was right.

Pain creates its own knowledge.

In 1802 a chemist named Luke Howard developed a simple taxonomy for the types of clouds in the sky. The shifting shapes of clouds had amazed and baffled humankind, but no one before Howard had given them useful names.

He had recorded how one weather event led into another and how to see the patterns. He called them *cirrus. Cumulus. Stratus.* He then broke them into subtypes that might be combined to create a complete vocabulary. He painted pictures of clouds in watercolor.

"Every cloud is a small catastrophe, a world of vapor that dies before our eyes," writes Richard Hamblyn in *The Invention of Clouds*, a book about Luke Howard's work.

I am a container for shapes that won't last. I stare at my internal formations as Luke Howard looked obsessively upward, trying to see the logic in the swirls and surges.

Doctor D, an osteopath, could do nothing new for my disease, because, as she said, there was no cure. I liked her honesty. Instead she prescribed a course of antibiotics and told me to get off the Tramadol and the steroids. I balked. Weren't those white oblongs the only thing holding me together? *No way,* I said. She said to try a lower dosage; there were studies that the drug might increase sensitivity to pain.

So I went off them, terrified for the wave of pain. Instead, my body felt almost exactly the same. I stepped into the naked world of pain on no pain pills. Later I got back on them again, when I needed a break, but I never take very much. It's hardly anything at all, and that's what using a pain pill feels like: a tiny sliver removed.

People without pain think there are pills for everything, but I have not found a pill that erases pain. Some shade it a bit duller, but if you're not treating the underlying condition, you're still stuck. Lost in it. Mired. Caulked. Frozen.

It took roughly five years of pain days to believe that the pain-free body had died. I need to understand that she is buried in photographs with my face, to understand that I am now living another incarnation of myself.

I have mental tantrums about this. I have Kübler-Rossed myself into fits of *no way, man,* whipping around the stages of grief, bargaining and denying like a Tilt-a-Whirl, jimmying locks and praying and buying potions and placebos and optimism.

I miss my former ability to think continuously. I want to wear a T-shirt that says, "Excuse my inability to process your spoken language. I won't be able to meet your cognitive expectations of me today."

My son is a leaping ten-year-old now, though he's still a snuggler. I still have to say to him: "Watch it, Mommy's in pain today," and I hate that. I hate that some fold in his memory is tucked with the sight of me wincing as he runs toward me with joy.

But he's learned that bodies contain mysteries, and that he might not know what another person is feeling, even if they look fine. He's learning to be careful with bodies.

I am a different person in pain. Not worse, just different.

If I were a pie chart, I'd be maybe 15 percent pain. The weirdest and most difficult thing I do each day is to try not to freak out about that. Instead of looking away, I have to study it, to know the way it creeps and shimmers.

Sometimes it wants sugar and a movie. Sometimes it wants work and concentration as a distraction. Sometimes it wants touch, and sometimes it wants the skin never to be touched again.

Pain is sometimes gray or turquoise. Sometimes it is shattered like lace or withered as an old tea bag. It is an anvil-hat or a cross of crickets. It is a body suit of burrs dipped in gold paint.

Pain has layers or levels, like a house. When I'm roaming around its ground floors, I can function and still get stuff done. When I go up toward the attic, I am pinned to the Now, the breathless present, the kind of heaven that Buddhists and mystics and kinks know.

I wish I had a safe word, but I do not.

I moved and got a job in Connecticut, hoping the escape from southern humidity would free me. It turns out I took my body with me, and the weather is here, too.

One day the August sky and the invisible cycle of disease sent shocks down my limbs and fogged my brain. I gave up on writing an essay and decided to just finish a short blog post about teaching. It seemed, at best, semi-incoherent, but then it went viral.

This raises the question of which woman is a better writer—me in pain or me without.

The pain-woman speaks in a pared-down voice; she is a dreamy laser. You can't tell her a single thing. She has room for only one emergency.

She has to creep slowly and hold onto the backs of chairs as she moves, but she has a strange superpower. She cares more about the vulnerable soft flesh of everyone than my normal busy pre-pain self.

She aches in slow motion for everyone's crumbling life. She sees dead bodies wrapped in skin, sees the present moment as death in reverse. She is in a kind of ecstasy—not the way we understand the word as joy, but the older definition in Webster's Dictionary: "an emotional or religious frenzy or trancelike state, originally one involving a mystic sense of self-transcendence."

And then there was a day, a quiet landmark on the couch: the first day that I realized I wasn't depressed because I was in pain. I realized my mood could separate from the bad news broadcasted by my nerves. I was okay in here, in terrible pain, but alive and watching it.

Pain explodes, over and over. It's also super tiring. And then I need food and sleep.

Later tonight I'll get depressed because I have lesson plans to do, and I want to be more than this ecstatic, shattered, staring beast looking at the swirls. But for now, I see swirls, and I feel the weather in my bones. And I am two bodies, and one is the history of me. And the other is a lava-lamp Ghost Girl with a new voice I have to listen to—no, more than listen to. She wants the keyboard, and she doesn't care about the life I had before she was born.

WELCOME TO THE KINGDOM OF THE SICK

When I am ill, only the kingdom of the ill is of comfort. The image of laughing, limber-limbed bodies with shining hair is not bitter because I long for it. It is bitter because it does not have anything to teach me and because it makes me forget the solidity of my own ground. I cannot aim for that bright country of the well anymore. It is barred to me, and as I hold it in my mind's eye, there is no room for crushing nostalgia. The taste is bitter because it is the taste denied.

What I learn is that the kingdom of the ill is a vast bedrock. We appear weak and reclined, yet we cannot be invaded or defeated. Look at us: We are unbreakable in our brokenness. We cannot be cured and are therefore invincible. We have dropped down the well. We reel in a slow-motion dance, treading where others fear to tread, continuing to breathe in the postnormal existence. We are the zombies, the undead. We are the good and bad witches, the double-sighted.

The kingdom of the ill is mighty and legion, and it is the borderland all bodies must pass through. And we have set up tents, encampments, and homes. We wave at you from beyond the gates.

When you have arrived, you have arrived. Welcome and blessings.

When you have arrived, you have arrived. Welcome and blessings.

When you have arrived, you have arrived. Welcome and blessings.

When you are aching, think of the vastness of the kingdom of the sick. Think of all of us here, feeling the most common feeling of the body in unfamiliar territory. The body feeling its own existence. The body uneasy, conscious, mindful, aware.

Dis-ease.

Feeling a roughness that polishes a moment, not necessarily to grant an easy enlightenment—not at all. Do not tell those around and outside that you are grateful for your illness, for they do not hear it right.

They will think that illness is a secret boon that delivers a greater intensity, a sheen that adds to the experience of health, and one that somehow delivers them back into the kingdom of the well. But that is not what you mean.

What you mean is "There is the secret door we all must enter, and I am entering it, and it is painted in luminescent colors that I am drawn to describe but cannot." What you might mean is "I am less afraid to die because I am dying."

What you might mean is "I see we are all dying in slow motion like flowers and without any diminution in intensity, and that is different from what I expected to feel."

I sit up in a shudder, my back lodged against the metal frame of the gate opening into the kingdom of the sick. I can still pass and carry my shape in the land of the well, though my dimensions are collapsing. Only the legion in the land of the ill offers comfort and beckons with the depth of this understanding. The ill are real, fully alive, such a vast and churning army, never ceasing. This is what I mean: they are permanent. The ocean of the sick with fevered eyes and bedrock has always been a stripe on the horizon, flashing pink and bright.

What I mean to say is this: A fevered look is not an unintelligent look, maybe not even a pleading look. It could be true that the kingdom of the sick does not even reach out its fingers to you to request and plead for your health. It could be that the kingdom of the sick wants nothing from you, because it contains you, because it is your alpha and omega, because it is your mother.

We are your living sunset, but we don't want to scare you with the sunset, which is your mother.

We are real, and only illness reveals the true bedrock of illness. It is not imaginary. This land is the most reliable and most vast of the human experience. I would make statues of the sick and dying, not to sob at the waste of sickness or death but at its normalcy, at the way the fluids flow out from these temporary containers. Illness is not a departure from the itinerary, not a battle, not a failure. It is the noble permanent out-breath, the quotation mark to close out the sentence.

THE ALPHABET OF PAIN

In her 2014 book *A Nation in Pain: Healing Our Biggest Health Problem*, Judy Foreman writes that chronic pain costs the United States "more than cancer, heart disease, and diabetes *combined.*" More than cancer, which we often view as astronomically costly because of the range of serious treatments and surgeries required for treatment. And more than diabetes with its many complications. Chronic pain, writes Foreman, "accounts for 42 percent of all visits to hospital emergency rooms."

The majority of chronic pain patients are women, and the medical establishment seems to have a hard time hearing or treating them. Instead many of these patients inhabit a spectrum of desperation. They have nervous systems that have been turned on in a very bad way, and they can't find the off switch. Our health-care system is very bad at treating chronic pain, and that affects everyone.

I am one of those switched-on bundles of nerves. It's okay. I'm still here. I'm not going to talk about the physical sensation. I'm after the meaning, the language of pain and its patterns. If chronic pain marks bodies, the bodies spell messages, books, libraries of possible solutions that are now as invisible as the pain itself.

Health-care costs in the United States continue to escalate, and a chief driver of those ER visits and expensive diagnostic procedures is chronic pain. A 2011 study by the Institute of Medicine estimated that 100 million people in this country live in chronic pain, and that number doesn't include children, people in the military, in prisons, or in nursing homes, places where pain is also legion. Pain takes over the central nervous system, blotting out the attempt to create metaphors to describe it or a numerical scale on which to rate it. But the burden of pain is also collective and systemic.

Our often-fragmented health-care system usually cannot see or treat chronic pain. Women's accounts of pain in particular are often minimized or ignored by physicians. Those in chronic pain visit specialists for the disorders and damage that might have started the pain and often shuttle between more than one specialist.

Imagine that the trigger was a back injury, but no visible injury could be seen on any scan. Other times it is a condition like fibromyalgia, migraines, or multiple sclerosis or an autoimmune disease, where the cause itself is unknown. If we are lucky, the doctors share test results on our various syndromes and injuries. Sometimes, if we are lucky, these doctors collaborate on treatment. We visit new specialists, try new therapies, and if we are very lucky and live near a major metropolitan area, we are referred to a pain clinic.

The desperation of all those human bodies in pain is horrible to consider alone without connecting it to meaning or thinking about the consequences. But the practical consequences might nudge us to a new way of seeing pain. We all bear the burden of escalating medical costs, so it must be said that the expensive task of treating chronic pain affects us all.

In the place where I work, my body is a problem because I use a lot of health care. I serve on the committee that discusses faculty benefits and compensation with the administration, and as we discuss cost containment strategies, we look at an anonymized list of "high-use employees," and I know that I am one, and that makes me feel guilty, somehow.

Every week, when I grab my binder and head into a conference room to talk with fellow faculty members and the administrators about how expensive we are to employ and insure, the administrators tell us about escalating health-care costs. They want to curb behaviors that are unwise and wasteful, they say, and the "overuse" of the emergency room is cited as a prime example of people utilizing health care in inefficient ways. This always makes me want to laugh out loud, as if these patients headed to the ER because they had nothing else to do on a Friday night, and the newest episodes of *Mad Men* weren't on Netflix yet.

I don't go to the ER for chronic pain. I have said to chronic pain friends, "I know that if this pain were suddenly visited upon someone without pain, they would be calling 911." People with chronic pain do go to the ER out of desperation. A spike in pain—or a grinding surge of pain—is terrifying, especially when one has run out of specialists, or the specialists have no new ideas, or one's general care doctor has no inspiration at all. Doctors who manage the syndromes causing chronic pain are rarely equipped to treat pain itself. Foreman writes that veterinarians in training get more education on pain management than doctors-to-be in medical school, and that only four medical schools in the country have a required course on pain management.

For immediate pain, patients are often given a prescription of opioid or nonsteroidal anti-inflammatory (NSAID) pain pills. Everyone's reaction to each of these is different, and moderating the body's tolerance to drugs is complex work. Many drugs work only short term, which is of no help to the chronic pain patient. And pain is a signal the body wants you to hear, a sign of danger, and it will work hard to deliver that signal.

Researchers know that once pain becomes chronic, the body's receptors to pain grow, which means that the body in pain becomes acutely sensitive to pain. While an olfactory nerve stops signaling a noxious smell, the pain and the body's pain signals amplify and often get stuck on high alert. This makes sense, because pain often signals impending extinction, so the body's survival mechanism is tuned to pay attention to pain even more acutely than to hunger or the need for sex.

Doctors uneducated about pain management or fearful of creating addiction can undertreat chronic pain, leading desperate patients to seek support elsewhere. Many people with chronic pain are afraid to take opioid pain pills because they fear addiction, though the vast majority of chronic pain patients do not develop addictions. They may become chemically dependent, but that is not addiction. But addiction and depression can bloom where a desperate person finds himself or herself alone in confronting pain, without the aid of a treatment team for advice and guidance.

Right now I'm in the kind of pain that would send a "normal" person to the ER, wild-eyed. Instead I take to Twitter and texting, to message boards and groups that save my sanity. I find myself caught in a web with other women's bodies and minds. We've been fused together, thankfully joined via the Internet, where we pool our symptoms and start advocacy groups and share diagnoses and treatment strategies.

Pain enacts itself in predictable ways and flows into the fault lines between all the other social problems one can imagine, mortaring the pieces in place. Those who are in chronic pain—again, mostly women—are viewed as unreliable, as an unwise investment, as a burden, as complainers, as unfixable. There are so many of us, women who are supposed to be caretakers, whose bodies have reversed the flow of care and said no, women whose bodies demand alternate systems of caretaking and new methods of healing. We also need new ways of seeing and naming pain.

I have been in pain every day for over five years. If I confess to a friend that I'm in pain, I realize there's no decent response to that comment. There has to be a way to end that conversation politely. The most common response is, "But you look great."

Sometimes "you look great" sounds like a simple dismissal. A woman's job is to be pleasing to the eye, so this comment might be meant as a comfort: I am still passing and fulfilling my most important role.

But other times this response buoys my spirit and kindles the embers of my vanity. For a moment I am not merely a puzzle to be fixed; maybe parts of me still work, or I can still project joy. Sometimes I'm grateful for any illusion or for the reminder that health and sickness, beauty and illness, can coexist. And "looking great" is also a comment on the mysterious gap between subjective experience and appearance. How can one be in pain and still walk around and function? Who knows?

The aversion to pain is as deep as the first nerve cell in the oldest organism. We would like to contain pain as a personal problem, a health-care issue for folders and privacy and sighing and "Get well soon." But if pain were not political, we wouldn't have torture and jails, both of which manipulate and use the body's instinctive aversion to pain to instill fear and compliance. We need to talk about the patterns of pain.

Chronic pain is not a missing limb or open wound; it is the essence of invisible suffering. In Kevin Brockmeier's novel *The Illumination*, characters in pain radiate light through their skin. I wonder what it would be like to live in a society like that, where our collective agony might blind us, or where the skin of the afflicted would shine as though they were ethereal beings. I wish I sparkled. I wish my pain made me beautiful, made me more noble, or was a fashion statement. Instead it is just pain, wordless and desperate for expression.

We all want chronic pain to go away—those who have it and those who don't. The massive gulf separating the pained from the non-pained can be summed up in one question: "Have you tried yoga?"

I reflexively have said the same things to others: *Oh you don't really want to kill yourself.* (I said this just the other day to someone).

Gluten free really helped me with inflammation (I know. Whatever. It happens to be true, but I shouldn't have said it.) This is both trying to get a handle on an unfixable tornado and, unfortunately, minimizing someone else's experience by implying I might be able to fix it. And we Americans—practical, fix-it folks—are particularly liable to stumble into this optimistic and ineffectual response. It's in the water.

I have tried and I enjoy yoga. But if you tell me to try yoga, then I will have to fight you. You will win, but I might nip at your jugular with my sharp incisors first. I might be physically weaker, but I am fierce, a fierceness born of frustration. What you don't see is that have-you-tried-yoga is a refusal to see this massive ocean and all the million ways I have tried to swim in it. I won't list them, but yes, I do currently include yoga stretches in my extensive list of methods for pain management. The scariest thing is that yoga is only pain management for a condition that is currently unfixable.

Our fix-it-itis is not a simple social gaffe but the evidence of a deep blind spot born with the help of the market. We are educated about illness by television commercials. Arthur Frank writes in *The Wounded Storyteller*: "Behind the hospital brochure and the commercial lies the modernist expectation that for every suffering there is a remedy." Cases such as those of chronic pain sufferers where there is no clear solution are mysteries, but "[m]odernity seeks to turn mysteries into puzzles, which is both its heroism and its limit." A puzzle like me that cannot be solved is a point of discomfort, a disjuncture, a black hole.

The chronically ill or pained body is a challenge to our notion of commercialized illness, writes Frank. In the typical television commercial for a pharmaceutical or over-the-counter treatment, "the good person is suddenly struck down, but suffering is bourgeois (for example, a missed party or sports event), the remedy can be purchased, and the only learning involved is where to find relief next time." This is why people recommend the market in all its forms to treat a mystery: pay for yoga, try this cream, buy some fish oil. My body is a discomfort, a burr in the hide of the marketplace itself, a reminder that not all pain can be treated with a purchase.

I passed a colleague on the path in front of our campus library, and she caught sight of my cane and winced.

"Are you hurt?" she asked.

I wanted to say, *Yeah, all the time*, but people see my pain only when I carry the length of metal pipe.

I told her I had rheumatoid disease. I vaguely waved my free hand in the air around my body. "It's autoimmune. Systemic."

"But it's under control, right?" she asked. She had somewhere else to be, as did I, so she turned and was walking backward, facing me but departing. I needed to let her off the hook, to make the complex simple.

I usually say, "Yes, I'm feeling good," but that was a lie, or at least a vast oversimplification. I shrugged and said, "As much as can be."

What I wanted to say to her is that pain is the essence of out of control. Our medical system cannot handle me and would like me to go away. Some doctors have given up on me merely because I wasn't an easy win for them. Doctors are people, too, and they want to succeed. It takes a strong and self-aware doctor to truly grapple with the treatment of a phantom that may not be fixable.

I am perfectly okay with the fact that I may not be fixable. I would like some help with pain management, which I currently do in sort of a slap-dash way on my own. I have a pharmaceutical cocktail prescribed by my primary care doctor that helps me sleep, because sleep is a kind of elusive magical healing place for people with chronic pain. I have rigged my own semi-workable sleep machine, but none of my specialists—rheumatologist, acupuncturist, endocrinologist, or chiropractor—deals with sleep or pain management. They each have a role to play, and I'm not a medical doctor. But I do my best to guesstimate and keep up on the research, which is my second full-time job.

The American Chronic Pain Association recommends an interdisciplinary treatment team for chronic pain patients, which would include nurses, doctors, social workers, and physical therapists. That coordinated care (oh how I desire it) would be amazing, but it often can't happen given the limitations of the health-care system in this country, in which cost-savings are squeezed out of health-care providers by decreasing instead of increasing time spent with and on each patient.

Ideally, treatment of chronic pain might begin by creating many more chronic pain clinics, places where people could go to seek help for pain that resists short-term treatment. Patients need a supportive team to assess what triggers are amplifying pain and what can be done to interrupt the pain cycle. This would save tons of money, prevent addiction, and reduce agony. Some pain can be treated surgically with nerve blocks, and others—the most frustrating cases for doctors—are those in which drastic interventions are not needed and won't work.

There is a pain clinic about 45 minutes from my house, but its website advertises a range of treatment for physical injuries but not chronic diseases like autoimmune disorders and fibromyalgia, primary sources of chronic pain for women. Another clinic's website seems to list a few chronic conditions, but when I click on the "other diseases," it takes me to a blank page. I read down through a few other pages and see that the focus is on spinal injuries and nerve blocks at the sites of specific physical trauma. In five years of daily pain I have never been referred to a pain clinic.

Because of the baggage I accumulated as a result of being a woman, I now minimize my own pain. When I go into my rheumatologist's office, they ask me to rate the pain, and I smile sunnily and say, "Oh it's about the same, a two or a three."

Eula Biss wrote an exceptional essay, "The Pain Scale," about the maddening nature of the pain scale. As she documents, I also struggle with rating my pain on a scale of one to ten, because I get hung up on what a ten might mean. Is it unassisted childbirth or dismemberment? I can't compare my pain to the worst pain imaginable. Plus, well, I'm used to handling things and making do. So if one is "making do," anything above one is what I really can't handle. Maybe this is not right. There's no time in the doctor's office to talk about these issues.

If I rate my pain a two or a three, do I mean that I thought about death only two or three times in the past week? I don't mean suicide, exactly, but rather the fact that death will be a solution to this. This won't last forever. Death is a comfort instead of the ultimate fear.

And then in my "two or three" there is also the wish not to be extreme in my rating, to be manageable. There's a *Seinfeld* episode (season 8, episode 5) in which Elaine fears her doctor is blowing her off. She gets access to her medical records and sees that he's noted she's "difficult." This is funny because it's also terrifying. I've seen the doors slam shut in a doctor's eyes when I have approached an appointment with raw desperation.

I have learned, through difficult experiences, that before an appointment it's important to get myself together. The worst thing to do during an appointment is to cry. It's important—for some doctors—that I display a sunny outlook, and others seem to respond better to a more muted and practical mask. Some doctors like it when I bring printed lists of symptoms, and others have reacted very badly to the same practice. It's important to look like I'm not needy, like I'm not trying too hard, and also not like I have over-researched.

When I was first diagnosed, my body still carried the vivid muscle-and-nerve memory of what it was like to be pain free, and I became feral and desperate to regain that level of functioning and physical experience. The abrupt transition into pain that arrived every day was like being buried alive. I went to specialists and cried. I felt entitled to health, to a cure. I demanded. I pushed for more treatment, and I pushed myself right off the edge of a health-care cliff. The specialist said that because he couldn't commit to one diagnosis, he couldn't help me. My primary person, seeing this disagreement with her own diagnosis, bowed before the important specialist at the university clinic and decided that a lack of clear diagnosis meant no diagnosis. She took me off the meds I had been on to treat the condition. I subsisted with no treatment until I moved, a year later, to a new area of the country and could start to rebuild my treatment team.

Doctors have been trained in environments of competition where cures and successes are prized. A doctor who can't solve or erase chronic pain might consider himself a failure. Or he might project that anxiety onto me, branding me a hysteric, a drug-seeker, and thus edge me out of his roster of patients because I represent the discomfort of his own inability to heal.

My next rheumatologist was wonderful, but she saw pain as equivalent to disease process. This is unfortunately an incorrect equivalency. In my syndrome and so many others, pain has its own existence. A rheumatologist is busy enough managing the disease process, but I need someone for pain.

I don't want to be a problem because I don't want to close off access to my current level of treatment. Not ever again. I am terrified in the doctor's office. I go in and I minimize. I shrug. I am bold in other settings but, as a result of pain at the hands of doctors, of dismissal, I have a kind of health-care anxiety that makes me elide what I know to be true for fear of being branded emotional, hysterical, psychosomatic.

The body in pain is a deviant body that defies expectations, refuses the easy boxes of sick and well. I am trying to figure out how to love a body in pain, or feel desire with a body in pain. The fibers of my muscles ache, and the muscles supporting the joints tense up around the pain. My skin often feels like it is burning, and that is not merely skin as symptom. That is the same skin that welcomes or repels touch. I have only one body to use, inside the doctor's office and out. My body remembers old embraces, skin-to-skin contact from before as well as now. Now there is a barrier between myself and other bodies: this pain.

Desire is a different substance now, a process requiring attention and effort. It is no longer a thoughtless release. Pain sex is queer sex, strange sex, wrong sex. Even in the comfort of a therapist's office, the assumption is that everyone *must* be having sex and must produce the requisite amount of desire. I have been encouraged and maybe even shamed a bit to get up to a normal level of sexual production because "sex is good." I agree with this, and it is important to feel connected to my partner in this way, but sex and desire are very complicated for people whose central nervous systems scream at them. Sex is a complex and fraught dance, an intellectually draining circus to run. After I manage to have sex, I often collapse for a few days from the effort of being in my body and sorting the signals of pain and desire. Yet I am continually pushed to conform. It's not that I don't want to have sex; it's that my partner and I are in the midst of tentatively creating what sex looks like for someone with chronic pain and her partner, and I don't see this image of desire anywhere—not in movies, not in what I read. As Lazy Rane writes on the blog *Guerrilla Feminism: Global and Intersectional*, "I believe that a body in pain, is a body which is particularly hard to love, and scarily easy to hate. What is worse, the pain can make this hatred of your own body seem not only reasonable, but inescapable, so blatant in its normality that it can take a long time to challenge your own feelings." Desire and love have to grapple first with reconstituting themselves in a body that has been altered to its core.

I sort of passively identified as queer before getting sick, though I hadn't been very out about it, but now I am constantly aware of being a queer body. My notion of myself as a conventionally performing "woman" has changed because I am less available to provide extra emotional effort in the form of friendliness, niceness, and emotional attention to others. I am more curt because I have to reserve my strength, and this necessity makes me more abrupt and less able to soften the edges of what I really think. Pain has hardened me into a different version of myself—me as if I were a desert, as if I were a house built by Frank Lloyd Wright. Pain changes the way I write and the way I think.

I usually dress on the feminine side, but this feels like a charade because I exist—for those I care about, for those who know—along the spectrum of contradiction, the but-you-look-great axis. I put on a dress I love when I feel worst, consciously manipulating others' views of me with regard to my illness. Sometimes I enjoy being "out" as someone in pain, and I dress to accommodate the pain. The way I shop for clothes has completely changed; I need comfort and nonbinding apparel above all. I've had to get rid of so many pairs of both cute and stomping shoes. Sometimes a cane is necessary for physical support but also as a sign and a signal to others that I am in need of a wide social berth, that I will be available to give you less in the way of attention today, and even as a sign that my cognitive processing speeds are lower today because of the pain.

Blogger April Penn writes, "Some days I can't tell the difference between pain that I have because queerness has remapped my body versus pain that I have because chronic illness has remapped my body. I will never be the same. That doesn't mean that I am broken, but it doesn't mean that others should project onto me how they think I should be 'fixed,' forced to see somehow that bodies are not panic-driven, that language without words is not fear." Not every experience of chronic illness or pain overlaps with queerness, but that in certain cases they do intersect. As one's body and one's desire radically change, one's world changes.

My relationship to myself as a writer and a worker has changed. I'm more in need of unplugging, the kind of unintellectual activity I have judged people for in the past. I watch a ton more Netflix and play games on my phone when I'm in a lot of pain. I used to avoid television and consider extra energy to be a reserve I had to dump into political work. I still participate in political groups, but my contributions are quantitatively much less, though I am also struggling to see my healthcare and disability advocacy as political "work." Sometimes I berate myself for not being up to the level of other bodies. Sometimes the language of the marketplace and the workplace get into my head, and I treat myself like a bad employee, someone who has to compensate for being "below average" some days and who, therefore, must struggle to pass and overperform on the days when I have more available energy.

As a woman worker, I have had to speak up to resist the expectation that I will be endlessly available. I wrote a memo a few months ago to various supervisors asking explicitly for disability accommodation regarding a certain category of job performance I had trouble with. This was awful for me, but necessary, a protection. A supervisor said to me in slightly concerned tones, "You've been *very* honest about your health condition." He was maybe trying to embarrass me or warn me; I couldn't tell. Honesty assumes, I think, choice. He was assuming I had the ability to hide, or that I had a decision to make. But I had no choice, and that lack of choice might be when bodies pass from normal into deviant, when the body leads and there is no choice but to follow. My body has become far more radical than my mind. It says no. It backs this "no" up by going on strike and becoming unmovable. It makes me rest. My body is forced to be brave in order to save itself.

People with chronic pain are at the whims of their flare-ups. They need flexible work hours and health insurance. Our economy makes it very unlikely that those two things will go together. I am a tenured academic, one of the few jobs in this economy in which I sort of control my time and also get health insurance and job security. Chronic pain visited upon a woman, particularly a woman of color with limited health care and income, is an additional crushing physical and invisible burden. Chronic pain is the invisible additional layer of work and stress as it accumulates on bodies, exacerbated by disparities in social support, income, access to health care, and access to decent food. I am a "person" at work, legitimized by my full-time role. Another good friend at work who has similar issues has to stay silent as she is a part-time worker on contract, and thus she would never know whether her request for accommodations would be the reason she might be seen as less productive and ultimately expendable.

Donna Haraway writes in her essay/mind-bomb "A Manifesto for Cyborgs" that a "cyborg is a cybernetic organism, a hybrid of machine and organism, a creature of social reality as well as a creature of fiction . . . The cyborg is a matter of fiction and lived experience that changes what counts as women's experience in the late twentieth century. This is a struggle over life and death, but the boundary between science fiction and social reality is an optical illusion."

I am a cyborg now, a strange, invisible, two-bodied being, joined in a way to my friend Elizabeth via two iPhones. We text dozens of times per day, on average, comparing notes. We check in because our similar illnesses have made us both feel alone. We both have joint pain, and we are influenced similarly by the barometric pressure and weather patterns in our geographic area. As we have become good friends and more and more honest with each other, we have begun to develop a specificity with language and geography that situates our illness in a real way with regard to weather, the planet, and our individual bodies. We both know a certain flu-ish, feverish feeling. We have pinpointed a certain crushing pressure, and its opposite, the agony of expansion as pressure rises. We feel humidity and a cold front in ways that we both, as writers, struggle to find the words for. We speak in the "royal we," queens of a nation with no known boundaries. When we name our symptoms accurately with words and confirm what the other is also feeling, we are doing research with our bodies as instruments. We text from respective couches but transcend loneliness and isolation. We make each other laugh despite being two bodies that are doing the opposite of what female bodies are supposed to do, which is to cavort actively while caretaking and consuming. We go to bed early. We read a lot. And we tell each other constantly that we are sane, that we are wonderful. Together we are making a path for sanity and dignity where one did not previously exist.

"Writing is pre-eminently the technology of cyborgs," writes Haraway, who imagines a "cyborg politics" that might rejoice "in the illegitimate fusions of animal and machine." In this fusion the dangerous binaries and dualisms of man/woman, human/nature and others might be overcome—though the path to that overcoming is not obvious. There's just a suggestion, Haraway writes, beyond "the maze of dualisms in which we have explained our bodies and our tools to ourselves. This is a dream not of a common language, but of a powerful infidel heteroglossia."

Chronic pain requires words to keep it at bay. My pain confounds me. If there is a path toward this heteroglossia, it is on the patient advocacy blogs and message boards, which provide a very real container for my body to continue and to thrive. Online communities pool our intelligences, research, and methods for coping into a multibeing organism that is the next stage of human evolution.

Chronic pain is invisible suffering. It would be a comfort if identity provided a solution, but it is only a metaphor, a tool. Treatment of chronic pain must see the sites where pain overlaps socially and how it becomes lodged in bodies. No one in physical pain imagines the virtual world as panacea. Our nerve endings cry out for reliable relief made flesh.

Chronic pain is a time-bomb detonating in millions of lives, a continual mystery to health-care providers who have 15 minutes to talk and a prescription pad as a simple fix. Our medical system shuttles the barely insured and underinsured from one specialist to another until many collapse and give up. What we need is a system that listens, first, to people who know how to write in pain's alphabet.

PRAYER TO PAIN

Pain needs no altar. It is a deity older than worship and recoils from abasement. Imagine pain's misery, in fact—it has no hands to help you up. It cannot stand to see your curled begging, wants only that it could absent its imprint from your form.

Pain is a tree, a rock, a mere thing of the universe. It is mottled kin to you, not supreme presence. Yet as a being it is as large as sentience itself and therefore cannot be other than a god, a cloud that is slightly bigger than all who are aware. Can you not see the way in which it enfolds us and defines us? Pain does not want to inflict itself. Its existence is probably its own greatest agony.

What pain desires is ritual. It wants old worship only in the form of regular attention: ancient abiding, the selection of a certain-sized egg, the bending of saplings, the tasting of the wind at certain marked times of the day. The only ritual pain wants is for you to build a scaffolding of yourself around yourself and above. The ritual is to know this scaffold as the double-helix from whence we come.

Pain is not other than you. Pain needs to see itself in the mirror through your eyes. Pain is more scared than you are; think of its existence. Pain needs you to look at it, sense it, count it, record it, recite its lineage in order to calm it, tell it the bedtime story of itself to make the fire into sense. I make the fire into sense.

Pain demands only that you unsnarl the necklaces: think of the tiny work of fingernails, the pulling of one link apart from another. Think only of the gentle motion of stacking spoons. Its only ritual is that you give it the dollhouse furniture of the gentlest minutes and that you soothe its forehead. Relent. You must look pain in the eyes like a child and tell it not to be afraid of itself.

II

SIDE PROJECTS AND SECRET IDENTITIES

MY ALTERNATE SELVES WITH PAIN IN SILVER LAMÉ BODYSUITS

My fictional selves are like Charlie's Angels or intergalactic pirates. They get so much done while wearing silver lamé bodysuits. Actually, there's no version of me that looks right in that kind of outfit, but I make up these women, and then they irritate me. I'm so *not* a super-hero. A few days ago I sat at my desk, decidedly un-silver-lamé, pretty much wrecked by 2 p.m. My hands hurt. My neck muscles knotted up. My elbows and shoulders throbbed. The joints in my toes stung. But I didn't even take physical inventory; I didn't have that much sympathy for myself. I wanted vengeance. Myself and I were going to have a little snit with each other. I looked at the little clock in the upper-right-hand corner of my computer's screen and thought, *Three hours. You're wasting three hours.* Three years ago that would have been a fresh half day, an oasis. Programs would have been designed, proposals and essays written, projects cracked open.

Remember that fantasy, caffeinated self? I saw a glimpse of her silver cape outside my window as she sped by. Up until a few years ago I had been relatively lucky, healthwise. Then after a thyroid problem, the symptoms of rheumatoid disease exploded full-bore, and I gradually pieced together my diagnosis: an autoimmune disease that attacks the joints. I had thirty-eight years of carefree and lovely mobility. Those years were wonderful, and I am so lucky I had them. Now I have some days of 90 percent mobility, but I don't take them for granted. Five years would seem like long enough to get used to a new situation, but my mind and my body both struggle with the burden of the people we used to be.

Emily Rapp's *Poster Child* tells the story of the experience and effects of a congenital defect that limited her mobility, requiring a foot amputation and multiple prostheses. She includes a vivid explanation of phantom limb syndrome, the effect of a mind that has already mapped its body and continues to signal the emergency of a missing appendage. Rapp explores deeply the effects of this challenge on her sense of self, how it changed every experience, creating new adaptations and permutations. She writes honestly instead of aiming to create a fantasy of unreachable saintliness. She doesn't push the "learning" and the "peace" of her experience, because it doesn't end. She also writes about the effect of constantly imagining the other versions of her life, the *what-if* bodies, the alternate universes in which she had two symmetrical legs.

My disease is not currently crippling, though when I look up the definition of the word "crippling" I see that it means "unable to move or walk properly." I can often walk, but what is a proper walk? I understand and appreciate, too, that some people claim the word "crip" or "cripple" as an affirmation of identity that includes disability. I wonder what my image of "cripple" includes, what it looks like. Maybe I'm afraid to admit it could include me.

And I've had years—decades—to take my body for granted. That past of taking myself for granted has birthed the silver lamé superstars. I still want a body I can take for granted, a body I can push, a body—the body of a twenty-year-old, I suppose—that occasionally needs sleep and food but bounces back stronger after a glass of water and a doughnut. I can't tell my brain to forget about what it felt like to be pain free. I will probably have longing toward those other bodies, how it felt to be them, for a while. Maybe for the rest of my life. But this phantom body syndrome, the fantasy version of myself, can easily take over if I let it. It's a video game of shame in which this body, the one I have, always ends up losing. I can't help but imagine a paradise in which I would get everything done that I felt I needed to do.

Those silver lamé women are fantasies, a kind of efficiency porn, two-dimensional cartoon bodies. I shake my head and clear my eyes of the flashes of silver, and I have to first name them, to realize they exist. They flit through my vision when I'm frustrated, when I want to throw down my purse and my keys and swear. I suppose everyone has to contend with these former bodies as they age. My breakup with my phantom selves is happening faster, sooner, so maybe I'm crossing a challenge off the to-do list. That's another fantasy, but one that's slightly more realistic. I have strange and powerful mental silver lamé abilities, and I believe powers develop to compensate for others that wither. I have to imagine new superheroes; on bad days I can wield my metal cane to trip my foes. As I squint for my close-up, the thoughts and ideas I have are sometimes foggier, but sometimes the plans I hatch are brilliant.

THE COUGH DROP AND THE PUZZLE OF MODERNITY

I've carried the wrinkled wrapper from a Halls Cough Drop in my wallet for over a year. Its presence is like a nagging tickle in the throat, as much an irritation as "Mentho-Lyptus" has been a cool balm. I feel a little wounded by this old friend. Since 2011, when Halls adopted the "Pep Talk in Every Drop!" campaign, the cough drops have been emblazoned with clusters of slogans designed to inspire a work-through-sickness productivity. I once took pride in my ability to muscle through physical symptoms. But chronic illness got in the way of that ego trip, and now anything can make me feel guilty about work. Even a cough drop.

I tucked the wrapper in the snapped pocket with my change so I wouldn't forget, or maybe so I'd think about what was so annoying about a wrapper that exhorts: "Don't try harder. Do harder!" Other slogans chirp: "Keep your chin up"; "Let's hear your battle cry"; and "Put a little strut in it." Each slogan is surrounded with the parallelogram shape of four Halls logos, and the diamond clusters repeat off the edges of the waxy paper into infinity like tesserae in a capitalist-bullshit mosaic.

Halls wants me to go to work when I am half-considering staying home. The cough drops—once my ally in the simply menthol act of reducing discomfort—now want to hear my raw throat produce a battle cry. They want my achy body to strut. This neutral and comforting presence has morphed into the coach in the corner of the boxing ring, cutting my eyes to drain out the blood, putting a towel around my shoulders and sending me back out there to get pummeled again.

The previous Halls marketing also emphasized productivity, but never in this overt, manic way. A 1982 commercial features Mr. Donoghue, a cop standing grimly in front of a bakery. A lady comes up to him and says, "Smell that fresh bread!" Mr. Donoghue replies, "Nothing can penetrate this stuffy nose!" The lady offers an opened package of Halls "With Vapor Action," and he takes a wrapped drop. Science-magic is unleashed as Mr. Donoghue is surrounded with foggy waves of vapor action, augmented with a kind of sparkly, twinkly, semi-computerized noise that sounds suspiciously like a favorite childhood toy of mine, a robot called 2XL that played eight-track tapes and asked questions. Mr. Donoghue looks skyward, touches his nose in wonder, and he can breathe. A day later he's got his own package, and he's looking hale and hearty.

Before I knew to get my allergies under control, I fought a case of the sniffles that often morphed into bronchitis or a sinus infection. I learned the hard way that mucus wants to turn into pneumonia. I bought dozens of bags of Halls. When I was younger, before I started to get seriously and permanently sick, I could shove my symptoms down into the corners of my awareness, power through with adrenaline and over-the-counter balms and then duck as the kick-back of feverish flu socked me in the face. I was always tempted to see how far my mind could push my body in the service of work. The blatant cheerleading/goading of the cough drop wrapper made me uncomfortable when I first noticed it, not only because it's so insensitive but also because it is such a clear echo of the way I talk to myself. I have been a labor activist since college, yet I am my own worst nightmare as an internal boss.

When I feel sick and decide I need a rest or, deity forbid, a day on the couch, I have to go hat in hand up to the boss's dingy office at the top of the stairs. Boss-Me apparently needs to inspire fear, needs to look with concern and doubt at Employee-Me's to-do list. Boss-Me sighs and says, "Okay, take a break, but I want you back up to full capacity tomorrow." I have been well trained.

Before I developed a chronic illness, I think it's fair to say I worshipped work—and specifically production. I believed that only work could make me safe in the world, could deliver me autonomy and the ability to choose to leave a bad personal or employment situation. I was a woman at the first generation of middle class in my family, fingernails dug into the faint edge of stability, and I felt as though every paycheck widened my grip on that ledge. I'd lived on my own with no money, which was fine and sort of punk rock, but once I had a child and had no money, dangling over the abyss and hustling for health care and food lost every ounce of its romantic sheen. As long as my résumé was developing, though, I would be okay. It worked: I got jobs because I could produce ridiculously well. For years after teetering on the edge of the abyss, I goaded myself into ever-increasing production partially through fear, with the sense that if I did not keep working hard, I might not have money for what I needed, or I might slip back into the scary place of not having enough or having to rely on someone else.

Developing rheumatoid arthritis and various other autoimmune collapses was my biggest experience with failure as a worker and, thus, with possible psychic extinction. I'd failed before, in jobs, at relationships, but each time I'd found lessons to extract and ways to be proud of the way I'd navigated a pivot. This time, I was altered. Every nose-to-the-grindstone method of maintaining my hold on safety had to be remade.

What's worse is that this is not resolved, because the entire foundation of my self-esteem—what I make—is still in jeopardy. I am a worker who must daily confront the abyss of nonproductivity. My head measures how much I do, but my body restricts what I do. I keep completed to-do lists and go over what I have done to assess whether I do what other workers do. Friends tell me I am a rock star of productivity, that sick I accomplish what two well people do, but my terror burns.

From the time I was young, the twin fear-based worldviews of Catholicism and the Protestant work ethic have dissolved like a cough drop on my tongue, the harsh internal monitoring systems that divide a body against itself, as imperceptibly subtle and magically scientific as Halls Vapor Action.

Dr. Kathi Weeks, a philosopher and author of *The Problem with Work: Feminism, Marxism, Antiwork Politics and Postwork Imaginaries*, describes the power of the Protestant work ethic, which "is advice not just about how to behave but also about who to be; it takes aim not just at consciousness but also at the energies and capacities of the body, and the objects and aims of its desires." The work ethic unwraps and consumes the body like a cough drop. A chronic illness also wants to consume the body from the opposite direction. If the work ethic seeks executive control from the top down, chronic illness throws wrenches in the machinery, stops the presses, throws up pickets and foments dissent.

But my struggle with my inner Mean-Boss didn't explain the level of unease that a Halls Cough Drop wrapper provoked in me about chronic illness. Its exhortations got under my skin enough to hitch a ride every day for a year in the change purse of my blue leather wallet. I took out the wrapper while cleaning my purse, intending to toss it. But I tucked it back in, uneasy because I sensed that even my own work ethic was not the heart of the matter.

According to Arthur W. Frank, author of *The Wounded Storyteller*, the marketing of over-the counter remedies has helped to define how we understand illness. Frank describes these commercials as an "insidious model of the restitution story" in three acts. First, "the ill person is shown in physical misery and, often though not always, in social default. Some activity with spouse or children is going to have to be cancelled or work missed. The second movement introduces the remedy . . . . Eventually the remedy is taken, and the third movement shows physical comfort restored and social duties resumed."

When I read this simple three-act summary, the phrase "social default" cut into me, because that is the state of illness. I have always felt guilty defaulting on my various roles, stepping out of personhood, and asking—begging—for temporary accommodations, promising to come back and shoulder my burdens. What's important, says Frank, is that the suffering and solution itself both become part of commerce: "[T]he good person is suddenly struck down, but suffering is bourgeois (for example, a missed party or sports event), the remedy can be purchased, and the only learning involved is where to find relief next time."

I have felt this reflexive need for purchased relief as a fog that surrounds me. Well-meaning people who learn about my health problems are thrown into discomfort, and the acceptable response these days is to offer an easy (if slightly insulting) solution: "Have you tried yoga? Have you tried turmeric? Have you tried meditation?"

First I tried to reply to each of their suggestions. Then I felt my intelligence being questioned, because as a responsible person I would look into every possible solution. Then I thought maybe I'd write a paragraph listing everything I have tried, sort of a sick person's résumé; maybe I could carry it in my wallet near the cough drop wrapper. Now, however, it's gotten to the point where I watch the advice-givers and their discomfort when I say, "I do all those things." They are trying to solve the unsolvable. Frank writes, "Modernity seeks to turn mysteries into puzzles, which is both its heroism and its limit." Chronic illness is a confrontation with everything modernity holds dear, and an "absence of solution makes mysteries a scandal to modernity."

I exist in the scandalous state of illness. I am someone who will not get well, an unsolvable puzzle. Modernism chafes against what twenty-first century bodies know through our incursions into postmodernism. We must chart new understanding based upon the body's lived experience, yet we still long for neat, easy solutions.

What I have learned, crossing the line into sickness and social default, is that I have to smooth out the twisted cough drop wrapper of modernity every day. I have to do this not only for my own psychic well-being but also because pain does not respond to the kind of mind-body separation that my worker-self has used her whole life. Pain is prehensile; something about its nature is to twist, like the delicate but tenacious shoots of a vine, so that it can embed and grab on. It ivies itself into the brick of my structure, weakening it. Pain twists me like the ends of a Halls cough drop wrapper. A few cunning turns transform a flat square of wax paper into a neat home for a lozenge. If I do not unroll pain, I carry it. The pushing and tension required to produce and produce and produce will, over time, destroy a person in chronic pain. The fear of social default will do the same.

I continue working because I must. I continue writing because I need to. Beneath all the pain, today has been another day of weather change, and my joints jar against the shifts of barometric pressure. It is a clogged, gray-sky, swollen-finger day. I am flat on my back and wrapped in the electric blanket, which twists around me and encases me. I am typing with the iPad almost vertical, held aloft on my knees, trying to press the letters while torquing my wrists as little as possible. I have downloaded too many handwriting notebook apps, trying to see whether the frictionless glass of the iPad's face will save my hands.

Once I believed that work could set me free, but I am learning that it delivers me to new locations within the machine. Now I believe in creative work independent of wages as a source of true deliverance, but I fear poverty beneath the machine. And the machine does punish those who fall into social default. Pain makes me feel inadequate for not being able to master it. Managing this pain is its own work, only this work must be done in the opposite way that other work is done. I must untwist the cough drop, smooth out the wrapper, and I believe that route will reveal things I do not yet understand.

FROM INSIDE THE EGG

I. RECENTERING

Pain's misfortune is a transparent goo. Within it floats a vibrant, yellow
sphere, my golden center, where a new normal exists. It is a secret normal, not recommended and definitely unwanted. Inside pain's shell, this
layered existence is a universe, one I can both take an explorer's delight
in and loathe. I am recentering. My bobbing yolk must not level itself
against a normal life, whatever that might be. That way lie misery and
shame. Consider these inner and outer layers to be simultaneously true
and yet in contrast to each other.

II. ON ONE HAND, THE "NORMAL"

Pain is my new normal, and I want to sink into
   the meat of it,
to push my fingers at its seams,
to probe its texture. I want to claim this little hammock,
to say, "Look! This too is a good home!
Strange and misshapen but still a living vessel!"
Some disabilities, like deafness, form cultures that don't
   want to be fixed but instead supported
and given equal access. Sections of the
   mental health community

have staked out a new existence
around the concept of neurodiversity,
　claiming their own normal.
Disability activists,
social justice activists, and anyone outside an era's
　definition of "normal"
have had to fight for representation
in the body politic's consciousness of itself.
I have to remake normal for my own sanity.
I can't live by listing what I cannot do,
what I mourn, what I miss. I will never:
run a marathon, do metal-working, crack walnuts, play soccer.

III. ON THE OTHER HAND, THIS IS NOT RIGHT
One danger of saying a disability is "normal" is that the word
becomes tinged with acceptance, as if we might
just let go the effort to fix it. Chronic pain is an almost completely
invisible emergency, underresearched,
and so to accept it is to acquiesce to suffering.
"Normal" is shorthand for the imaginary
location where all our Venn diagrams overlap.
Normal is a reference point for the idea of equality,
a fiction of expectations, useful because it allows us to
demand fair treatment in relation to that mean.
Normal is also a vague and squishy category,
a homeland that we can ignore
that only gains meaning when we leave.
Does someone with a disability desire to be "normal" or to pass?
I pass and then I fail. At home, in private, I collapse.
When I confess my pain, I am letting out a
specter that makes other people unhappy.

IV. "NORMAL" FOR ME AND
RECENTERING, YOLK AS THE LEVEL

"Normal" in my case may mean not having to fight to
   hide the symptoms of excruciating
or annoying physical or mental pain. A 2012 survey found
   that 47 percent of adults
in the United States carry some form of chronic physical pain.
   Add to this near-majority
the anguish of sadness or a chronic mental condition,
   then add addiction,
then add the tension of racism and sexism and the
   waves of social exclusion,
and this is our normal: a thin smile, a slice of sunshine,
a series of masks to hold our collective and separate agonies in place.

I have not always been in pain, but it looks as if I
will be in some form of pain from here on out.
   That's not to say that I am
negative or have lost hope for cures or treatments,
   but rather that I am attempting
to come to terms with it, to recenter my life around
   my own experience.
Yesterday I read an article by a favorite female writer on
   the value of doing
manual labor with your children. The photo showed
   a fistful of hay, golden rays grasped in a glove,
backlit by a barn. I wished I could bale hay with my son.
   He was downstairs playing video games.
I sat down on the couch with my coffee, bobbing inside my egg.
Stop thinking about the crisp, fall air and baling hay.
   Stop it. Just love your coffee.

You cleaned the bathroom sink. Then you cleaned the toilet.
  Then you went for a
hat trick of functionality and removed the flecks of silver nail polish
  from your fingernails.

V. BUT PAIN IS AN EMERGENCY SIGNAL

I could define pain as "normal," but that
does not change pain's essential feature,
which is a nerve signal of danger.
Pain should not be normal, expected,
within the range of okay and taken-for-granted.
In every case, it's not okay.
It's a sign of undertreatment, underresearch,
social neglect, or biological wrongness.
One study found that 53 percent of pain
patients had their pain undertreated.
Medical personnel and the elderly both
viewed pain as a "normal" part of aging
rather than something to investigate and solve.
I am not adequately treated for pain.
I have come up with my own treatment plan.
I see several specialists but am rarely,
if ever, given strategies for the pain itself,
which is my primary complaint. I quickly stopped
complaining in order not to be perceived
as a "difficult" or drug-seeking patient. Now, if anything,
I drastically underreport the pain I am in,
a common conundrum for women with rheumatoid arthritis.
Chronic pain technically has no positive
utility for the individual body,

but I believe this pain has meaning for the
larger body politic, the community.
The causes of autoimmune syndromes have not yet been knit together,
but the alarm addresses our toxic world, reacting to the stress
doled out to the bodies of women and children in particular,
the way we carry and echo inflammation,
the violence within and beyond families and economies.
Our silent pains are the stretch marks on physical bodies
stretched beyond their carrying capacity.

VI. A JOINED VIEW, FROM INSIDE THE EGG

The level of energy and functioning I have now would have been an abomination to my twenty-five-year-old self. She looks outward occasionally through my eyes, aghast, and I have to tell her, again and again, where we are now. What is the word for this egg-land, this layered existence? It matters because it is both wrong and fine. Pain is not "my battle" or "my gratitude" but my egg.

And then there's the matter of the eggshell, delicate but incredibly strong. We who are in pain do not grimace or lie down on the sidewalk. Maybe we learn our carrying capacity as a way to keep the cogs of society functioning. Maybe we hide the pain to preserve our own pride and autonomy. When a person confesses to being sick, she is seen as less reliable, less capable, and therefore less of a person within the social and production networks of the well.

Pain is a social contagion. Across cultures, fear of addiction to pain medication and belief in stoicism reinforce ideas about keeping pain to one's self. Stoicism fights depression in one way even as it feeds it in another. Pain makes people wince in displeasure, so it's hard to be a bummer. It's equally difficult to smile and nod and lie.

Many cultures value stoicism as an appropriate response to pain. Pain is seen as an external expression of a system out of balance that will right itself eventually; patience will cure it. One cross-cultural study of pain responses found that men in Latino cultures avoid seeking help for pain because the admission would challenge a notion of machismo or strength as a man. Within the African American community, a legacy of slavery led family members to the acute awareness that expressing their suffering was disrespectful to elders who had been through so much worse. Chinese Americans may also display stoicism because of a connection to reputation in the community and a respect for the social status of the doctor. Many cultures also express fear that if they confess pain, they will be prescribed pain medications that will lead to addiction and therefore weakness, a drain on the family and community.

The study cautions against generalizing these cultural thumbnail sketches. Instead, caretakers and doctors are urged to ask questions:

"How do you manage your pain?"

"Are you afraid of becoming addicted?"

Only one doctor has asked me how I was doing with the pain, and she was a particularly caring general practitioner, not one of the dozens of specialists I've seen over five years. I've been prescribed all kinds of pain pills, the kinds that fog the mind without delivering relief or that abrade the stomach, damage the liver, and quickly fade.

We are primitive in our methods, and the nervous system is a mystery.

VII. TO LIVE MY "NORMAL"

Pain is the signal that something is amiss, wrong, or bad.
Here I am on the couch. I had to call in sick to a meeting. I
am waiting for a call from one doctor, and I know
I have to go to another doctor this afternoon.
And all throughout my body,
the danger signs and red lights are flashing:
abnormal, amiss, wrong.
I am living in that red glow, but after five years of it, I have
managed to make a transition in how I see this glow.
I don't mean that I live in peace but that the glow has taken on nuance.
I first went through a solid year of panic at how
horrified I was to be in pain all the time.
I had pain, and then I had mental pain *about* the pain.
Gradually, over the following four years,
I began to understand that that red flashing light of
   pain is not a crisis. I have an incurable disease.
That doesn't mean that I as a person am abnormal,
   dangerous, or amiss. I still go into that panic rejection
of pain almost every day, but most of the time
I can separate the two strands of discomfort from each other.
I want to hate the pain without hating my life for having pain in it.
I have to constantly remind myself that the pain
   is not a sign of failure
and that I am no longer living by the standards of normal bodies.
For me, this pain is perfectly unsurprising.
Now I chart pain's nuances; I feel a weather front,
   a stress ebb, a muscle ripple.
I must attend to the details of pain's ecosystem that the
   world does not understand.

VIII. AMISS, AWRY; HAVE YOU TRIED YOGA?

Somehow we feel we deserve the pain. Maybe
we have not adequately looked into imbalances in our lives,
have not adequately tried to heal ourselves.
This is the bite when someone suggests yoga or swimming,
the implication: *If you tried harder, you could fix it.*
This response joins two strains of American spirituality,
both the New Thought of practical healing through the mind
and the Christian notion of suffering
as penance for bad behavior.
The first historical definitions of the word "pain"
in the Oxford English Dictionary define it as
"punishment; penalty; suffering or loss
inflicted for a crime or offense."
The second is "the punishment or suffering thought
to be endured by souls in hell, purgatory, etc."
The real danger for me is that I often take on the world's
negative judgments of pain as well as the pain itself.
If I am in pain, I must be bad, wrong, amiss.
This creeps in especially when I'm tired or run-down,
and especially when my pain overwhelms me.
Physically, pain provokes sensations of panic and danger:
my chest tightens and my breath shallows
when my brain realizes my body is in pain.
I have to get beyond the idea of my brain being scared of my body.

I lie here, trying in a half-hearted way to respond to work emails.
I'm getting stuff done, and then I'm resting, by the
    light of this red flashing light,
and although there is a glare, this is my life.
This is *my* normal, and my body is well within the
    range of human experiences.

I am not *abnormal*. I am on the bell curve and part of the human
community. Some of us have pain, and we are still people,
exploring the full range of what it means to be alive.

I don't feel like I'm fully abled anymore. But I'm not disabled.
Or am I? I have regular physical impairment, including manual
dexterity and mobility, but I rationalize, slip down, say, "Who
doesn't?" "It could be worse." I have cognitive changes mostly
due to sleep loss, but I blot those out because they depress me. I
have participation limitations, energy limitations, all the
hallmarks of restriction. Admit it: This still makes my
breath catch, as if I could fight to get out of a cage.

So what kind of creature do you turn into when your eyes adjust? How
does one's skin grow translucent and beautiful after evolving in a cave?

Like a transitional object, pain has becomes a friend of sorts, or at least a
companion. Not an easy companion. Even with a difficult relative, there
is pleasure in the knowing and patterning, the attempt to understand
one with whom one lives, the lure of almost getting it. I come to know
this pain that surrounds me because I have to keep my hate in check.
Pain is my very flesh. There's no "brave battle" here. I refuse to be at war
with myself. I just am. I am layered with another presence as if draped
in a transparency drawn on in red marker, inhabited by a being that is
of me and yet separate. Its cycles overlap with mine, its irritations are
triggered by my actions, yet its logic is mysterious. It cannot tell me
what it wants or needs.

Right now, five years in, I am at midlevel pain, a plateau where
a new normal can be built. Humans are incredible in our
adaptability, our ability to dig homes in the mud, to decorate

with sticks. When my fingers are on the keyboard,
my brain flips a switch, and the pain recedes.

There's a theory about the "gates" of pain in
the brain that shuttle signals,
but I can't look it up right now.
I can do only certain kinds of thinking in pain.
I can think through a keyhole.

It's important for me to know this pain. I sit and feel it. In the
overlay, my fingers bulb at the ends and the knuckles. In the comic-
book version of me, there are red slashes up the back of my neck,
a line of festering cratered sores up the right side of my spine,
and my fingernails peel back. Imagining the marks of this pain
makes me feel better. If my fingernails were peeling off, I'd take
a moment to collect myself. I might take a break and not feel
guilty. If I were in a comic book, I'd feel less shame because my
werewolf nature would be a superpower. These layers are invisible:
the yolk that surrounds the bright, yellow-orange sun of my
thinking mind, my strange nerves, and my still-beating heart.

CUPCAKES

What does my son think when he sees me lying on the couch under the green blanket, feeling sorry for myself but more than that sorry for him? He just got home from fourth grade on this September in 2013, and he's playing video games, and he just had an argument with the neighborhood kid, and I can very easily imagine staying on the couch like this for hours.

There are no cupcakes waiting for him. When I berate myself for my mothering, it usually involves a vision of cupcakes.

I'm lying on the couch in a fever, but not even the kind of fever where you get chicken soup and time off from life. This *is* life, this collection of autoimmune diseases that comes and goes. It's come and gone every day or week since he was six, and now he's almost ten. He's seen me hobble around with a cane. He knows I have something up with my joints and something wrong with my thyroid. But now I don't care about those things. I just wish I could get up and do some kind of—what, cupcakes? Fall centerpiece arts and crafts with him? Things I never do when I'm well? Something. Instead it's screen time and brain rot, and I am overwhelmed with what to make for dinner.

It looks like I'm doing nothing here on the couch, but I'm excavating shame, dipping down into visions where I am a bad teacher and a mediocre mom. To compensate for this fear, I throw myself into work whenever I am able, probably overcompensating with the emails and the meeting and exceeding of deadlines and goals. The time that other people spend drinking, watching sports, getting their nails done, playing Candy Crush, or cooking fancy meals, I spend sick. It's my hobby. When you're rock climbing, I'm sick. I have lots of good patches. I'm just in a bad patch. And I'll be a good worker for a long time. I am like Neo in *The Matrix* but with pain and discomfort. I work smarter and harder in short bursts of brilliance. Rah rah, go Team Sick.

The recent blood test results seemed worrisome but in a way that I couldn't interpret, and I put in a call to the doctor today and didn't hear back, and I didn't hear back either from the other doc who ordered the tests. So I am on the couch wondering what those numbers mean and whether they can fix it and wondering why I have to wait for three more weeks to see a new specialist, because my last brilliant specialist had to close her practice. At least I have insurance. If we were Canadian I wouldn't have to do that little simpering dance of gratitude for what is a human right. But anyway.

I didn't feed the bearded dragon lizard his chopped vegetables. I need to put a load of clothes in the dryer. And I have deep suspicions that my insights about Ben Franklin's *Autobiography* won't seem very insightful to the honors students in my seminar tomorrow. I responded to a few student emails and slept for an hour. I worked for six hours this morning, but it never seems enough.

My son comes upstairs, and I tell him out of guilt that he needs to get off screens in a half hour, and then he can help me figure out what to cook for dinner. His stepdad, who is so helpful, is working tonight. My son says okay, and I go back up and lie on the couch and start to cry because he's so good, and I have a half hour before I have to do something practical.

I text a friend who also has autoimmune stuff, and she realizes pretty quickly that I'm losing it, so she calls me instead, and she makes me laugh. She asks, "You want to make your son *cupcakes*? Do you actually ever make cupcakes?"

"No," I say. "I guess I must be a bad mom."

"You're a great mom," she says. "Mothering and baking are not actually the same thing."

"I feel like crap, and I am afraid of everything," I say. When I have a fever I get this thing I call fever doom, and I can't think straight.

"I get that too," she says. "Tell your son to make a PB&J, and he'll be happy and fine."

My son comes upstairs in his little polo shirt, and I start to cry and I say, as I always say, "I'm not upset at you, buddy. I'm just not feeling good. You know that, right, buddy? It's my joints and my thyroid."

He nods. "Let's go to the library and get Chinese food," he says.

"Okay," I say. "Good plan."

We go to the library, and he checks out a Pokémon game and a video and a book in a series he likes. Both inside and outside the library, he scales concrete walls, slides down banisters, leaps and jumps. On the way out of the library, a guy passes us on the walk, looks at my son leaping in midair between two concrete blocks and says, "I wish I had his energy."

"Definitely," I say.

My son and I get Chinese food, and on the way we talk about why it's good to buy from local businesses. I'm not sure when this conversation started, maybe a month or six months ago, but it's been on his mind lately for whatever reason, so we often list the local businesses we buy from. Tonight we talk about why it might be better for the family running the Chinese restaurant to work for themselves rather than having to send their money to McDonald's Corporation.

Okay, I think. He's getting vegetables in his Chinese food. I can't do fall centerpieces but I can do social justice economics.

We drive home and unpack the Chinese food, and I stare at the unwashed dishes in the sink. This is it: the sink, and my hands and wrists burning as I grab the first glasses to put them away. So. Tired.

But we keep on, and I tell him to get out the soy sauce for him and the fish sauce for me.

"Eat the broccoli, okay? You need it to get strong," I say. And the fever hasn't gone anywhere, and I pour him milk, and he tells me to come downstairs and sit with him.

"You can type on your iPad, Mom," he says. I can't see much; it's like the edges of my vision are gray, but that makes things simpler.

Tonight I will tuck him in and go right to bed because extra sleep helps, and I hope in the morning I will feel better and get calls from doctors, and I'll drink all my special potions and do my special vitamins and relaxations and be the best mom I can be. And he's already the best son. And this won't be cured because not everything is a princess story, but—but what . . . . I feel the urge to write "That's okay," but it's really not okay. It just is.

I never excelled at the domestic arts, but I made up for them in hustle. My son and I used to bake a very simple kind of sugar cookie, and the point of those cookies was the icing, the cutting out of weird shapes, the art projects. Often the cookies themselves would go uneaten. It was the making, not the perfect product. I am not staggering under the weight of a previous generation's baking expertise or longing secretly for a cupcake myself. I don't really even like cupcakes. Maybe it's Pinterest, which I'm not even on anymore. I deleted my account because it was making me feel bad about myself.

I'll admit it: I don't like to bake things.

A few months later, with another dip in health, I am in my therapist's office, and I am crying about my mothering and baked goods again. "I should be a better mom. I should be making cookies." I have been trying to support my new reality by following more disability activists on Twitter, and as I think about what I've been reading, sitting in the soft chair across from my therapist, I have an idea. "Wait," I say, looking at her. "That's really ableist of me."

I realize that to be a mother, my expectation is that I have to be active, capable of physical challenges, in constant motion with my body, reaching and straining and hanging things, and shopping for supplies to make complex constructions. I realize that I don't see much of the emotional work I do, much of the repetition and the quieter acts of constant attention and care. Instead, I evaluate motherhood purely through the eyes of a crafty photo spread or an exhausting educational field trip, both of which are completely beyond me on most days.

I'm setting myself up to fail by comparing myself to some crafty marathon that has nothing to do with what I believe about love.

I drive home from the therapist's office, crying, fighting off the edge of pain, trying to maintain a slim grasp on the insight I had while sitting in her chair. That evening, despite a short temper, I am buoyed by the kind of desperate edge that makes me want to do one useful thing to spite my own life. I go to the health food store and buy gluten-free chocolate chips.

I don't bake partially because I don't do eggs or wheat or a thousand other things, all in an attempt to calm inflammation. I've tried breads and cakes and all that stuff, and I've bought the mixes and the cookbooks. I do them sometimes, but sometimes I get tired just thinking about the chemistry of foods.

Somehow that night I do make cookies, spooning the egg replacer into a little dish, mixing with water, adding it to the tapioca-rice-xanthan gum flour. I waver at the counter, telling myself to just focus on the next task. I enjoy the baking in that moment, because it is at least something. I can't do email, and I can't think, but I can do this. For some reason this feels like it gets me more credit in the mothering department, which is supremely weird.

My son tells me he doesn't want to help with the baking, but he comes in to peer into the bowl. He asks for a lick, and he can eat all the batter he wants because there's no raw egg to make him sick.

I drop the cookies onto a cookie sheet, and he sits on the couch staring into a screen. I bring him a spoonful of batter. The timer dings, and then the cookies turn out good even though they are gluten free. When they are warm and just out of the oven, I bring him some on a little plate, but he wants only a few.

He's actually not that into sweets. He's not a baked-goods kind of kid. We both like the idea of cookies and cupcakes but find their sweetness cloying.

A few days later, I'm out of granola so I eat the remaining cookies for breakfast. I wonder what will remain in my son's mind as the shorthand image for mother-love.

My own snapshots of mother-love have nothing to do with baking. I see my mom collecting moss and dirt to make a little garden in a plastic bowl. I see her hands tapping the steering wheel of the car as she drinks a Tab and sings along to the Eagles, happy to be on the road with her family.

I wonder if my son's rock-solid knowledge of mom-love will be the smell of animals, the shells of horseshoe crabs we have collected, the skulls and bones to encourage his interest in nature. Maybe it will be my weakness itself, my cane, or the smile I am able to muster that glows with what I know is pure affection no matter how I am feeling. I cannot know what will stand in for cupcakes, what will hold the smell of mother-love, but I know it will not have icing.

AMOEBA GIRL

The pain creature that overlaps with my body is born anew each day, a colorful double image superimposed with shimmering edges. She and I are strung together with the most delicate meniscus of surface tension, the membrane of an amoeba constantly evolving. She nibbles at my edges, though I try to hold her in check with the wavelike motion of my cilia, the silver line of to-do list tension that keeps me afloat and a step ahead. But I can't stay ahead of my pain-sister, and she enfolds me in the salt water of my origins, unable to stop the storm surge of the ocean where we evolved together. We wanted to be sentient. We wanted to feel. And this is the cost of our evolved nervous system.

Sometimes the slick amoeba skin of pain swallows me, and I toss my head and say *no* like a fevered child. I want to be like other bodies, but I've only known past versions of my own. I review the snapshots of nerve-splashes in a spring-green album of physical nostalgia. I want to be what I once was.

What was I? I lie on the couch and sing the prayer of my skeleton's history. Even as I remember brown, strong limbs and the delight of running roadside with stretching stride, I catalog the troubles where bone met bone, before I had a shining membrane of pain.

That skeleton had the thumbprint of trouble: a left hip that clicked when I extended my leg; bunions on the base of both big toes that grew red and large as plums by high school, even though I wore only tennis shoes. In junior high I sat with a heating pad on my aching knees to soothe growing pains. I spent my twenties pursuing endless gynecological solutions to pains I now know were centered on my aching left hip.

Japanese potters who work with the philosophy of *wabi-sabi* include a flaw in their creations to highlight the nature of this material world, marked with imperfections that are the thumbprint of beautiful asymmetry. I was born with two relatively harmless birth defects, a hemangioma in my right shoulder that was removed to prevent profuse bleeding, leaving a scar the length of my palm and a lumpy ball of scar tissue that pulls my neck out of alignment. I would not know my shoulder without that ladder of rippled flesh. A chiropractor examining my X-rays after a car accident pointed at my stacked spine and told me I had a few vertebrae fused together in my lower back. "You're supposed to be a little more tall and flexible than you turned out," he said with a chuckle.

This collection of stout stakes, hammered and jarred by a few car accidents and whiplashes, has been nonetheless strong and storm-worthy. It was eminently healable, up to the point when my immune system surged against itself, overtook, overshot, began purely by accident to attack, like a pot boiled to bald, like a song sung to a hoarse whisper.

Dear strong skeleton, dear irritable immune system, dear girl-body bathed in the midwestern greenery of petrochemicals and nitrate-soaked well water, dear inflammation gone awry, dear logical response to a series of triggers forming their own mysterious music, a personal periodic table of the bones and elements that made me. Dear logic. Dear mysterious crullers of code, dear alphabet of genetics inherited from mother's and father's family tree, irritable skeletons from both sides that gnarl together, curling around my joints like the clever vines of morning glories.

Here is the dilemma, Amoeba-girl: your skeleton, that strangely evolved pointy thing, is your mode of locomotion, but its edges burn.

Pain is the cost of your movement. I lie back on the couch and acknowledge the Pain-Body Amoeba Girl, the one who remembers life before bones, the fragile one who aches, the one who bursts through the membrane of my denial, cool, hot, surging with chemicals and an old language I do not understand but that my body seems to remember.

III

MY MACHINES

THE STATUS OF PAIN

A friend at a writing conference asked me how I was doing. I said, "Pretty good, all things considered."

"That's good," he said. "All I see on your Facebook page is 'Pain, pain, pain.'"

I gave a half smile and a knowing shrug to get away from the conversation, but my brain buzzed with distraction, embarrassment, annoyance, and a bit of curiosity. That's all I'd managed to leave as tracks on his brain: pain? Was he razzing me in a failed attempt at flirtation or maybe trying to be sensitive in a backhanded way?

Then I began to worry that I'd set up an inadvertent Wailing Wall on social media, even though I'd tried to do the opposite. I had made a conscious decision to post as little as possible about my medical adventures with rheumatoid disease and Hashimoto's thyroiditis.

Sure, I needed to vent. After scrolling past enough pictures of people's dinners, rock-climbing feats, and dogs, I felt compelled to put a bit of myself into the maelstrom. And sometimes I wanted to share that my life was also part of the big picture of life, even if it was posted from flat on the couch.

The last thing I wanted to become on social media was what I felt like in real life: pain, pain, pain.

When I was in college, a young woman in philosophy class told us that she had chronic pain from ulcers. I couldn't fathom it. Pain, like stubbing your toe, but *all the time?* Wouldn't that drive you to the brink? She was beautiful and a campus athlete, and I began to revere her from afar as some kind of saint, which was the reference point I had for unrelenting suffering: that it ennobled.

Lucky for me, I had exactly twenty more years to live my lovely, normal life, filled with sex and sports and walking and soccer and sleeping late and hardly ever having to fill prescriptions. My body could swing and shake and dance for hours. Eventually my immune system revved up into crisis mode when I was in my late thirties, which catapulted me into rheumatoid disease. It's systemic, autoimmune, and incurable. My joints hurt pretty much all the time.

Since then—in case you're tempted to share with me your quick fix—I've tried everything, and I manage stuff like a pro. Supplements, exercise when I can, a new diet, medications, acupuncture. I work it like a job, and I have to say I am as responsible as one can possibly be in caring for this very needy pet. But although pharmaceutical company commercials want us to believe that new drugs make life better for everyone, the drugs for my condition don't work all the time, and they don't erase pain.

Pain itself is a weird experience, but you get used to it. It's as tiring as parenting a newborn. It creates so many interesting conundrums and challenges. You can imagine it as adding a *World of Warcraft* addiction or a constant remodeling of one's kitchen to your already busy life. That's what it's like: a weird project you have to manage in addition to everything else you already have going on. A weird project that will never go away. Imagine remodeling your kitchen for the rest of your life.

People who don't know pain think it is really depressing. This makes sense, because it is the core biological imperative for preservation of one's existence: avoid pain. Run, in fact, from any mention of it.

When I post on Facebook about being in pain, or admit to pain in a casual face-to-face conversation, I read the winces in the emoticons. I feel and see the edges of my friends' mouths pull back in grimaces of displeasure, winces of agony, as if they themselves are feeling discomfort. As if, in mentioning it, I am the one hurting them. They don't want to talk or hear about pain. But they have questions, and they are embarrassed to ask. Some friends do ask, and I have loved how they listened as I tried to describe it. I feel very cared for in those moments and immensely relieved.

It's hard to figure out what to do with this pet Pain if I can't post pictures of it on Facebook. It's not going anywhere, and it makes other people uncomfortable, which adds to my own discomfort. Not only do I have a physical problem to deal with, but I also have to feel guilty and watch that I don't inflict thoughts about pain onto other people. People want to tell you their grandmother cured her osteoarthritis with cactus juice. I've done the same for different difficulties, responding with vague clichés about "what makes us stronger" when friends have lost parents, marriages, jobs, and medical battles.

It's hard to know what to say. It's easy to say the wrong thing.

Sometimes it's harder to watch someone we love suffer than it is to suffer pain one's self. I can't do anything about this pain aside from doctors, walking on the treadmill, and eating turmeric and fish oil like candy, but at least I can *know* it. That's what causes anxiety for others, I think, and for me: pain is unknown and unfathomable.

I decided to read through a year's worth of my Facebook posts to assess whether this friend's comment about "pain, pain, pain" on my Wailing Wall was accurate. Because I love Facebook, I had hundreds of my own inane status updates to click through, mostly quotes about writing, teaching, books I loved, political activism, and events on my campus. I had posted links to articles on fighting racism, pictures of my family, jokes, laments about my dying car, and a photo of a squash that we'd kept on my kitchen table for over a year because my son drew a face on it with a permanent marker. I posted about getting solar panels, my love of the cartoon *Adventure Time*, and many thoughts on the Affordable Care Act. I posted ideas for imaginary band names and jokes about *Star Wars*, as well as an update on what happened when I spilled a full can of seltzer on my desk. I posted about the sport of soccer-tennis, a trip to Hong Kong, kayaking, and the zombie apocalypse.

Throughout the whole year, June 1, 2013 to June 1, 2014, I discovered six posts about my illness. Three of these were not about my own situation, but instead links to content created by other people: a graphic about national awareness day for rheumatoid disease, a link to a survey about rheumatoid disease, and a link to a book about coping with chronic pain. The remaining three posts gave updates about my own health situation, all within a few weeks last summer in which I had a thyroid crash and was having problems with my energy levels. One was a simple apology that I was having trouble returning emails in a timely fashion. The second: "When I have the energy, I'm going to write about finding the energy to parent with an autoimmune disease."

And the third: "It turns out that giving up caffeine after a 22-year habit is actually not that big of a deal if you have RA. I have learned this morning that my pain tolerance and my pain levels are both so high that a teeny little caffeine headache barely registers. It's kind of cute, this little chemical headache trying to act all important."

Two posts for the entire year had mentioned "pain" by name.

In that last post, I injected some humor as a way to sweeten the subject and not drag my friends down, and also because it's one of my own coping methods: I have to laugh at it. At the same time, I was trying in that status update to give myself a little credit. I do have a high pain tolerance, which I've known for my whole life. People in chronic pain are often desperate for a sense of how others might experience their level of pain, because they would like to know whether they are merely being overly sensitive or whether they are dealing with something that is as epic as it feels.

This is all complicated by the fact that pain research shows that a chronic pain sufferer's nervous system can get activated and become permanently on alert, so that everything does feel like agony. The question is epistemological, as most questions seem to be: how would this pain feel to another person? Pain is not an abstract essence. It is an experience, a process.

My friend might have been exaggerating, but I believe his comment, and his memory of the "me in pain" that I'd shared on Facebook, meant something, despite the fact that it was factually incorrect. Pain is searing, and it creates an emotional connection. Expressing pain affects others deeply, creating discrete and uncomfortable memories. One expression of pain, and that is what he remembered. This, too, must be keyed into our species' survival.

When I thought of this friend and his own online persona, I happened to remember most vividly a few honest posts he'd made about his own troubles. It could be that empathy burns those associations into our brains, and that we vividly remember the strong emotions that are drawn forth by the agony of others.

The question, then, is whether even a few honest statements about our conditions become what people see when they think of us. If we are vulnerable, will people automatically associate our whole beings with those moments when we are at our weakest?

My awareness of my health image began well before my friend's comment, and I'd also been consciously checking myself. I felt embarrassed after I posted more than one thing about my health because an administrator at work, who is also a Facebook friend, said, "You've been *very* honest on social media about your medical issues." He said the word "very" as if I'd done something scandalous and unwise, or as if I were into an odd hobby like sticking goldfish up my nose. Or as if admitting to rheumatoid disease were akin to posting a picture of myself doing a keg stand. He's one of those administrative types that make you feel as if you might be in trouble for everything.

After his comment, I got a little paranoid and decided to post less on social media about my pain, partly out of vanity: I didn't want to be depressing. I wanted people to see me as someone who had more going on in my life than pain. I wanted to be seen as sexy, lively, cute, funny, and relevant. Smart. A thousand other favorable adjectives to please my ego. So maybe vanity won over honesty, or maybe I was trying to condition myself to focus on more than the pain in my joints.

After I'd made the promise to myself to craft an idea version of myself, a witty, well-read, upbeat figment of my imagination, another friend said, "I noticed you haven't been posting stuff about your health on your page. You must be doing well. I'm so glad." I wanted to tell her about my continued troubles, about the complicated nature of invisible disability, but I said nothing. We hugged and rushed off in opposite directions to our next work responsibilities.

I have gone back and forth about what risks I take when I publicly acknowledge on the Internet that I am sick. Or that I am me plus a sickness or however I might want to describe it to make myself feel better on a particular day. For a while I thought sharing would actually protect me, because I figured that the more people knew, the more they'd be required not to discriminate against me. But this is a whole other legal and medical privacy conundrum. I know, ultimately, that the social protection of sharing outweighs any of this, because I stumble slowly into networks that will be truly supportive when the chips are down.

I know that the data I post on social media might be used for specific marketing purposes and is public in a way that might impact me in the future. I can't be denied insurance for a preexisting condition under the Affordable Care Act, but new methods of discrimination are always being hatched. Still, this condition is already listed everywhere in my records, so I'm not safe anyway. I can't maintain a cagey fear of anyone finding out about my health-care issues. Pretending a big part of my life doesn't exist only makes me feel insane and ashamed, as if I have done something wrong that I need to hide.

For that reason I have decided to be "out" despite the consequences, but I have to remember that I am able to be vocal about a few conditions in my life due to social privilege. I'm a writer, so if someone does discriminate against me on the basis of a health issue, I can put it up on the Internet in a reasonably coherent narrative. I'm an activist, so I would know how to make a stink about it. And I'm a tenured professor with a decent income, so I have the flexibility and time to write, the ability to have a flexible schedule that works around my illness, the support of colleagues, and the ability to be relatively safe from health-related discrimination at work.

Off and on I have felt that having an invisible disability was a burden I needed to crack through, and I wanted to normalize it, to bring it into conversation so I wouldn't feel the stigma of having an unmentionable to carry around. I needed people to know what was really going on in my life, because the pressure of trying to pretend to be normal was more exhausting than being sick. I needed my coworkers and friends to adjust their expectations of me. I needed them to know what I was up against so that they might understand when I said no.

Before I got sick, I said yes to everything, anything anyone needed me to do, and after I got sick, I had to stop it. Putting my reality on Facebook was a way to train myself and others to deal with my new normal.

Or did I just want sympathy? I admit, at my weakest moments, that I did want that. But I also wanted to benefit other patients, which is a major motivation for people who post information about illnesses on social media. Most patients are willing to share their social data to help patients like them, even if there are privacy risks involved. Hence, the link sharing. A survey found that 33 percent of adults use social media to find out about medical conditions and "to track and share symptoms." For that function, I would sometimes post questions or comments to a series of Facebook and blog comment boards where patients crowdsource information about new treatments, tests, medications, research, and side effects.

At base, I wanted my friends to understand me, including this new little wrinkle in my life. I wanted to be "out" as a person with rheumatoid disease because being quiet about it added shame and loneliness to a host of other problems, mainly the pain.

It's hard to know exactly what I want in response. Sympathy helps a little, but not if it directly morphs into my friends' agony and discomfort. Instead, like sharing haircuts or publications or travails about broken cars, I just want them to know and to have known, so that they can form an accurate and honest picture about me and who I really am. That's intimacy, I suppose, and it seems to break down the wall that anxious sympathy erects.

And it's true: I do have chronic pain. But I can name your imaginary band in two seconds, and I have a thousand books you should read, and I'll send you a link to a great news article, and I think your dog is really cute. And I do have a lot more going on than lying on the couch. It's just that right now . . . I'm lying on the couch.

PEERING INTO THE DARK OF THE SELF, WITH SELFIE

I take pain selfies. These pale olive ovals float in the grid of photos on my phone, each a record of rheumatoid arthritis flared up and receded. In these images, my face seems to glow from the aftereffects of concentration and stillness. I am often lying back, my eyes lidded at half-mast, head tilted upward. With neither a smile nor a scowl, these faces are as close to the naked self as I might ever capture.

So in trying to free up memory on my phone and delete a few images, my thumb hovered above the trash can icon below one of these portraits. Why save a record of past pain? I assume that most snapshots are meant to capture loveliness or call to mind pleasures past, but so many serve to mark time and place, to say *I was here—at this monument or this sporting event, this wedding or this funeral—and my small piece of this large story matters.*

My pain selfies mark time, though I haven't collected them consciously. Instead, a secret urge overtakes me after a day or a chunk of hours on the couch. I surface from pain and want to see myself. Or I want to record that I have reached a mile marker on an invisible trail.

I admit that past pain is a strange thing to record when present pain will always arrive to compete, and future pain can be safely expected. Pain selfies seem almost masochistic, a collection of low points I should let go of. Yet I do not erase them.

I take regular selfies, too, maybe prompted by garden-variety vanity or maybe as part of a vast arts-and-crafts movement. Sometimes I look nice by accident, and I pose myself next to a window, raise my phone and try to catch . . . something. My smile is usually all wrong—too goofy, too tight. I tell myself I want to find an arty author headshot to use when it is requested, but I also want to document myself as looking better than the image of myself I carry in my head or heart. I've seen me at my worst, and the best is an interesting aberration that might actually push against my critical self-image.

These regular selfies sometimes document the rare burst of me feeling sexy or proud of myself. *Look at me lookin' all good.* The selfie serves as a kind of bookmark when I'm feeling down. In capturing a burst of self-esteem, a regular selfie can act as match to light the self-esteem of future days when I'm unlit and withered.

These images are also a way to find pleasure or appreciation amid days and weeks where I often feel as if I'm all hands, with a blur of incomplete projects, unmade dinner, and unfolded laundry piling up around me. A selfie pulls me out of the tedium of days to allow me to narrate, to say that even here, amid the tasks, I am alive for future versions of myself to remember.

Posing myself as my version of attractive is an accomplishment, I think. I'm normal looking, and I've grown much more fond of my face over the years, but any American girl who's gone through adolescence has felt the sense of being passed over and discarded as inadequate, nice except for that nose/those hips/that whatever. Our teenage fairy tale told us we were beautiful if a modeling agent discovered us in a crowd, at a mall, while buying ice cream, picking us out from among the crowd like the hand of God.

The pretty selfie is sometimes semifictional—or maybe aspirational. There is nothing dreamy, easy, or blurred about my personality or my face with its sharp eastern European edges and its stress-induced squint, but with the right filter I can look self-confident, spunky, and composed. I can look arty or silly, and I am framed the way I want to be framed. The square of the picture's edge announces that for this moment, this woman was all she needed to be. Once or twice a year I will post the pretty selfies on Facebook, when I'm feeling less than pretty, to get the boost of my friends telling me I am beautiful, because my friends love me and because they are kind. Needing that should not be such a self-centered or foreign concept.

The selfie is supposed to mark our particularly narcissistic age, but self-portraiture remains mysterious and even sweet to me, a flashlight peering into the self's darkness. Sometimes a regular selfie is a question seeking an answer. I wince at the ones in which the question in my eyes is too naked: Am I beautiful? More, even more than this: Can I succeed in making the edges of myself appear to meet? Can I be unragged?

And no matter what the urge, I think selfies are an arts-and-crafts movement, a populist act of composition and artistry, like weaving pot-holders or trying one's hand at gardening. With the filters and cropping and editing available at the swipe of a thumb, our simple apps invite us to see the mundane as sun-lit or shot through with shadow and thus to find the beauty in the mundane. We used to have to wait for the record of our camera work and pay by the shot, but now we can check, erase, check, erase. The phone on our camera is another eye.

And not all selfies are beautiful. I take some that are strange, with weird lighting in odd, in-between moods, and they ask the question: what does this moment mean, where I am at the edge of something I can barely feel? It is also lovely to document the face we do not know fully, the self we cannot fully know yet is our own, at a moment when we don't have words for how we feel. That, I think, is the beginning of all art.

These pain selfies come from an urge that has a question and a sense of self-esteem at its heart. I am looking for something connected to dignity, and I am curious.

The pain comes in waves and builds from a background pain to a trap that closes shut around me like the jaws of a whale. With it comes the pain-doom. I close my eyes and trace the failures this pain has caused. I have let people down, I am a bad mother, a bad employee, and an even worse housekeeper than usual. (If you have been unfortunate enough to closely study my kitchen floor, you would know that the bar is already set pretty low.) In pain I am useless to the outside world. I lie on the couch, wrapped in an electric blanket, submerged in the signals from outraged nerves. Once again, as with the regular selfie and the regular self, I have a hard time charting exactly who I am supposed to be and what the self in pain should do or look like.

Pain's song sounds like this: *What is this? What next? Who am I? What does this mean?*

The pain throbs and pulses like the magnetic lights of aurora borealis over a frozen landscape. I try to intuit the logic and feelings of the pain. What makes pain tick, and where is its weather steering?

Eventually I give in and move with the pain's motion, which can take hours or a day. I relax in the muck and fade in and out of a kind of transcendence. I cannot let go of the pain, but I stop fighting it. I ride with it, though that doesn't stop me from checking my phone and texting my annoyance about this pain to friends who will respond.

And then, hours or a day later, I am tossed back up on the shore of my normal life. As after a flu or Emily Dickinson's great pain, there is a formal feeling. Colors shine with hidden significance. Time catches on the wonder of itself.

I reach for my phone because I am curious about whether I have molted or been transformed by my journey. For those hours I have been separated from concerns about packaging and presenting my experience. I have been so far away that I wonder whether the container of me still exists. I don't try to look terrible. I don't want to document agony nor do I want to seem to look well. I simply want to regrow my skin and have a package again. Here I am, on the first day of this next part of my life.

I find the outward signs of my face in the phone's window: the wild eyebrows, sad eyes, and the sharp shape of the lips. The vision of my own face calms me down as I see that my features are miraculously still in order. I do not try to look sexy or cute. Pain pushes even gender out of the way, even vanity, even the hopes of looking like someone else. In some ways, pain returns me to childhood, my eyes to the naked, peaceful orbs of animals.

Thrasher skateboard magazine often featured a section of the gross, spectacular road rashes and horrible injuries suffered by skateboarders who bailed on tricks and destroyed themselves. When I dated a skater, I guiltily loved this section of the magazine, the grim pride of the wrecked, the fascination with seeing how the world can bash a body. There's also the sense of an invisible story with each image; nobody would send in this kind of crash-brag picture if the damage had not been healable. So the picture itself is testament to the happy ending, even if the dude now walks with a hitch in his step.

The pictures join the skaters to a tribe in an initiation ritual. The photo is testament to an achievement: I survived this. I am hardcore.

I, too, am hardcore, yet I am bragging to no one—maybe besides myself. The tribe of chronic pain sufferers does not demand this proof of a scourge that often leaves no mark. The mark, therefore, is on my face, and I can see the journey written there.

When friends tell me, "Well, at least you look great!" I know that my skin belies my immune system's relentless attack on its host. The pain phantom leaves no visible marks until much later in the disease process. For now, there is almost no visual way to make this real.

So I think I need reminders of those pain flares to understand the full scope of what I live with. I need private signposts to remember that what I feel is real. And maybe this is what any selfie does. Maybe it reminds us of all the places and feelings to which we have been anchored in time and space.

Although I share many details of my life in text, I don't think I'd show these images to anyone else because they don't make sense without a caption, and that caption is not yet written.

The image itself, in proclaiming an essence of pain, would ask for a kind of pity from the viewer, because the event and occasion is "pain." What I want to say about pain publicly is very different from what these images capture.

I like writing about pain because it is an intellectual project. I have control. An image of me in pain—or in the aftermath of pain—would require strenuous correction against an empathetic response. I don't want people to say, "I feel bad that you are in pain."

Empathy is an act of the imagination that grows from a gut-twinge of sympathy, a notion that I would not like to feel what that poor other person is feeling. We override our own flinching instinct to ask what another person's suffering might feel like.

Empathy can be troubling, too, if the imagination is done with a kind of arrogant certainty. A well-meaning person—particularly someone who is used to knowing things—might confidently assert their ability to empathize. But pain, I am learning, is always a question to which there is no answer, and that is the experience.

An expression of empathy or sympathy can feel like a door that has been closed instead of opened. When someone says, "I feel your pain," that may mean, "I actually know your pain because I can imagine it." Here's the thing: I don't understand my pain. It is wilderness. It is the open back of the wardrobe that leads to Narnia.

Susan Sontag writes in *Regarding the Pain of Others* that pain was once viewed as "exaltation" in a religious sense rather than "as a mistake or an accident or a crime." Sometimes I feel that in writing and revealing pain, I am revealing wrongness. The human instinct of empathy winces with another's pain, packaging the mystery of pain into an assumption. If I were to caption a selfie as "Pain Selfie," the word "pain" would trigger a wince and an "I'm sorry." But what I actually mean to explore is the weirdness, the inscrutability. And, too, the exaltation.

If I were ever to show anyone these pain selfies, I would show them reverently, as things of beauty, the way others post pictures of themselves after hiking long distances up piles of rocks to stand at a summit and look out across vast valleys and gulfs of silence.

That's how I think I look in them—stunned at a landscape that only I can see, exhausted from crossing it, wiser in some inward way for having crossed, and unable to say what I have seen.

I've shared ridiculous self-portraits, including pictures of my head wrapped in a "Terrible Towel" to cheer on the Pittsburgh Steelers in a Super Bowl. I take self-portraits with my face askew, and I think they are funny. My face is mobile and stretchy, and I like to bug out my eyes and look ghoulish. I share these with friends who know the inanity of my face when animated.

But I want to protect this other woman, the pain woman, who is not yet able to speak like my normal self. The images of her are private notes toward a story. When I take pictures of her, I am pulling my face up out of nothingness.

I think this is why I photograph her. As I capture her, I am trying to love her in the way one might welcome a long-lost relative, a woman linked by blood but whom I barely know. That woman is dazed from a long journey and needs to be guided back to her life. This is also an exercise in empathizing with that woman, myself. You would think that having empathy for the self would be easiest, but it is a challenge, because I use her eyes to peer out at the world. She is my instrument, and I forget every hour that she is flesh.

I need to love this self in pain, because I am so hard on her, and quite frankly, she disappoints my expectations. She knows that I would, on some level, like her not to exist, and so I constantly have to make up for that. I want her to be different. I want her to get more stuff done, to energetically call her son up from the basement where he is playing on his Xbox and immerse him in astronomy or whittling or some enriching Montessori-inspired activity. I want to be better than my pain, but I cannot will my way through it. I have willed my way through so much pain in my life, and now I have come up against pain that is bigger than my will.

The pain selfies help me reckon with an understanding of this. There is a woman who has been mowed down. Don't hate her as she goes under, I tell myself. See her beauty and her realness. Take a photo to remember her.

As critic and writer Anatole Broyard was dying of cancer, he wrote: "Every seriously ill person needs to develop a style for his illness. I think that only by insisting on your style can you keep from falling out of love with yourself as the illness attempts to diminish or disfigure you. Sometimes your vanity is the only thing that's keeping you alive, and your style is the instrument of your vanity. It may not be dying we fear so much, but the diminished self."

I am trying to capture the face of my new love, and I'd call this necessity rather than vanity. I am seeking the best light and the best side of the woman who does not have to pretend she is not in pain, the one who has let herself go under and goes on trying to fall in love with herself.

AUGMENTATION

My cane is made of two metal tubes, one fitting inside the other and held in place with a screw collar and a retractable spring pin that allow the user to adjust the cane's height. The cane makes a snickering shuffle-click with each step. The nested metal cylinders slide slightly against each other and then rebound against a metal pin that holds the collapsible tubes in place. When I drop the cane or smack it on accident against table legs, the metal tubing echoes, a high-pitched clink, as if the cane were longing for something far away.

The cane has a hard rubber tip meant to provide traction in varied terrain. Up close, the tread of the tip looks like a target with three concentric circles. I note with some strange satisfaction that the tip is worn down in the back from scraping forward against the pavement. This reminds me of a similar pattern at the heels of my shoes, and I find I want this: to leave my mark on the cane.

The cane has a black, foam handle, and at the very end of the handle dangles a black loop of braided synthetic cord. I find this cord somehow very dorky and annoying. I have not removed the loop because I slip it around my wrist when the cane is in danger of falling out of my grasp.

But it is true: I have a tiny corner of my brain devoted to annoyance at the style of the lanyard loop at the end of the cane. The cord is not any different from lanyards clipped to nametags at conferences. Maybe it's not the lanyard itself but the industrial hoop and eyelet of metal that affix the lanyard to the cane, or the metal closure that turns the cord into a disproportionate figure eight. I suppose the lanyard is equipped with this metal hardware for the sake of durability. And the cane has been very durable and reliable. What annoys me, I think, is that the cane is the opposite of hand-crafted. It is mass-produced and without any of the superficial, stylistic nods toward fake hand-craftedness a middle-class, twenty-first-century American like me has come to expect in her purchases. When I look at the cane, I know I am not special. I know I am connected with everyone else who picked up a cane at the drugstore because their mobility was threatened in a long-term way, a way that signals disease, limitation, or death.

When I recognize all it has done for me, I have to admit the cane was a very good deal for $19.95. I don't need it for months at a time, and I sometimes forget I even own it, but when I need it, I need it completely. I treat it with a mix of dependence and resentment, a very teenage combination.

I bought the cane in 2011, about six months after I began to feel symptoms of rheumatoid arthritis. My doctors told me that the sharp pain in my joints and the fatigue and fevers were hallmarks of an autoimmune disease. My disease had arrived with much fanfare and diva behavior. This disease would not be negotiated with, and it wanted accessories.

At first I did not even imagine I would need a metal stick. I did not admit to myself that I had even seen the rack of canes, and yet I knew it was near the back pharmacy counter where I waited to pick up my medications. I believed fervently in these medications and waited for the chemicals to return my strong body to me. It took me a long time to understand that for these diseases, the chemicals do not work like a biological Etch A Sketch. They manage what cannot be erased.

I returned to the pharmacy to fill a prescription for pain pills. The rack of canes bristled in my peripheral vision to the right of the pharmacy counter, near the bedpans and other large equipment for managing bodily decay. I would not look directly at those basins and seats with metal tubing and plastic receptacles in understated blue boxes. But the hardware had entered into my awareness in a new way. I never had considered my body a target market for these poles and slabs of plastic. Now I had to turn away from them actively, as if they might pursue me.

I had once skimmed and glided and dashed over the planet, but gravity began to adhere me to the earth's surface in new ways. My ankles and feet began to suck and not be team players, and my knees began to wobble and have attitude problems, and my toes began to be awkward and bitchy. I needed something like an oar to help me power over the pavement. I began using other random, long objects. I leaned heavily against counters and tables, hauling myself up stairways by the railings.

The idea that I might purchase a cane approached in two phases. First came an expanse of watery dread, the weepiness of not wanting to go where I had to go. And then, as with most transitions, I got sick of being mired in my own swampy resistance and found the cold delight of a decision, even if it was an unpleasant one. Being able to choose augmented mobility made me feel as though the disease had not stripped me of control.

I drove to the drugstore with the same kind of grim and desperate determination reserved for a breakup. I was going in to shoot a horse. I was going to murder the version of my life that had not accounted for canes. I was going to be super-adult about this because I needed to get stuff done. I would not combine this with normal purchases like tampons or shampoo. I would not bribe myself with candy, which would have been a violation of scale and perspective. I had mental energy only for this one private transaction.

I limped to the display rack and considered my options, from black and wood-handled to silver and hospital-like. I wrapped my fingers around the cool surface of a black metal cane printed with a pattern of tropical orange and purple flowers. The print seemed jaunty and fun compared to the others. I knew on some level that a fun, flowered print would not distract me from the substance of the cane. But I had hope that maybe the cane and I could get along. Equally as important, the print might protect me from whatever I imagined others might wonder or believe about me. I thought if I could communicate that I was a jaunty-cane girl, I might not seem so dire or patientlike to others.

I hefted the cane in my hand, put it on the ground, and leaned my weight onto it. I took a step, and the cane and I were immediately joined. It was so easy: with one tube of metal I felt more sure-footed. The pressure in my problematic left hip released, and my balance steadied. It was a length of pipe, and yet I felt in some ways the same intimate connection I have had a few times in my life when I've locked eyes with a future dear friend or partner: hello there, you who will get past all my feints and ruses, you who will know me as deep as my skeleton. Those who help me get through the day are not always flesh. And so I realized it loved me in its own way, and in my own way I would fight with that love, push it away, chase it, scorn it. As I walked three-footed up to the front register, the cane clanked like medical hardware but felt like flying a flag of surrender.

I paid for the cane and went out to my car with it. I flung it into the front passenger seat. I closed the door, cried a little, and told myself this was a temporary thing, this life-with-cane. I drove home and composed myself. I was a single mom at the time, and I needed to relieve the babysitter and present this object as normal, helpful, and fun— not scary. My son was six, and I imagined he might enjoy a two-foot, handled, metal thing because he loved lightsabers and swords. But he furrowed his brow and saw the cane for what it was, a foreign presence describing his strong mom's weakness.

A few days later we visited an evening fun fair in the parking lot of his grade school. I parked and pulled the cane from the trunk to clomp through the cotton candy fog. He ran ahead, scowling back at me across the dark asphalt.

"I hate that. Put it in the car," he said. "Everyone is looking at us."

I called ahead to him, explaining in a patient mom-singsong how all bodies are different, and each one is fine the way it is. His lithe, tan legs galloped and scissored his body away from me, and I could not dash to chase and catch him. I could not bend to gather him up and hold his warm body close to mine.

A few days later, the ache calmed. I left the cane near the door and stepped gingerly on my own, relieved. In the months that followed, my knees and ankles regained stability. Here's how it goes: There are months where I can forget about the cane entirely, and I can sometimes even jog for brief moments and dash to catch my son. I can pass him a soccer ball. But I always feel it. It's not like a sore muscle where the ache comes hours afterward. Right in the moment of use, the synovial pockets say *no*. I walk on the treadmill and walk the dog to stay active, but the dashes and feints of recreational soccer or the mind-clearing hum of a solitary run are no longer options for my skeleton. It's not that I am afraid to hurt myself but that I am entrusted with taking care of this system in which my soul hangs.

I have gone as long as six months without needing the cane. I walk easily when a complex combination of diet, stress relief, exercise, supplements, and medication calms the inflammation. After each bout of difficulty with walking, a fairy-tale part of my brain says *take that* and *I beat you* and shoves the cane into a corner, as if the metal tube itself had caused my weakness, as if by hiding it I could erase my need.

In the fall of 2013 the pain in my left hip flared wildly, but I couldn't find the cane. It had been awhile, and I'd banished it, thinking I'd reached a safe plateau away from it. I rummaged in the front closet, engulfed in old-shoe smell of moldering leather, looking for the glint of metal. I twisted awkwardly, sitting on the ground because squatting strained too many vital joints. And I was half-weepy, with the narrowed focus of a flare that has run ahead of me. I reached behind an umbrella, and my fingers contacted the hollow metal tubing. I lifted it out and set it on the wood floor sharply. Here was my strength, and I treated it like family: often disparaging it, but returning to it for support. That month I needed the cane every day, and I applied for a temporary handicapped parking tag.

During that month my son ran through our kitchen and grabbed the cane from me. He parried an attack from an invisible opponent.

"It's your ninja weapon!" he said.

He used the word "your." I called it "the cane." Not *mine*, as if the possessive pronoun would make a difference in terms of its permanence and its power over me.

And he had forgotten to hate the cane, or it had become part of the furniture in our lives. He was three years older. He knew mom was sick but not dead, still mom.

I didn't feel like a ninja, but for a brief moment I imagined the cane as a superhero asset, a cyborg augmentation that might make me something more instead of something less.

I clomped slowly into doctors' offices for X-rays and MRIs to determine whether there was a bone deterioration as the result of RA, or whether the answer was a familiar medical shrug. I waited for results, knowing in any case that there would be no easy fix.

I crossed paths with a coworker one morning as I navigated to my classroom building. I had my cane in one hand, and with the other I pulled a rolling cart full of books and papers.

A walking body approached a walking body. The cane has made me aware of these subtle, bipedal interactions, which are full of unconscious signals. We avoid eye contact but nonetheless judge speed and trajectory by the direction of the other person's gaze and position of the limbs and torso.

The cane seemed always to break that pattern, to require a glance down and then a glance up at my face. My coworker's eyes widened slightly, taking in the cane and hesitating, looking up, giving me wider berth, and attempting to make eye contact. I gazed back with a slight smile, as if to say thank you for the extra regard. In a vulnerable state, I realized that the cane was as much signal and warning to other clumsy humans as it was physical support. It itself was language.

Another day I was caught in the entryway to the English building amid a clutch of long-limbed undergraduates clomping and flitting around me with their massive, swinging backpacks. Pain tends to make me muddled and wavery, and I felt off balance. The cane spoke its silent letter "r," the shape a kind of growl: rrrrrrr. I whacked its tip on the cement floor so its metallic snicker resounded to call attention to the potential danger: *This woman cannot walk well. Do not knock her over.* The cane acted as a shield, speaking for me, saying what I was too tired and overwhelmed to say.

People who know me as energetic and bipedal see me with the cane in the halls and stop short, stricken—even if they've seen the cane a few months prior. "What happened?" they ask, eyes wide. I am tempted to say "skiing accident" as a private joke, because most of these friends do not live with chronic invisible illness. They see me as well. I deploy the signals of general normal movement, eyeliner, a nice outfit and earrings, a smile and conversation—and they forget. How could they not? They cannot understand that skiing and running are no longer options for me. I've told most of them I have rheumatoid arthritis, but what might this term mean, even when I say it is autoimmune and incurable? These things are thankfully incomprehensible to a body without these sensations. They tell me I look great, and then when I'm having a truly awful run of things, the cane reminds them of all they cannot see. The cane is a stoic messenger at odds with my smile, and they are hushed by its industrial anonymity and its power.

During that same flare-up, two of my students limped into a class with their own temporary mobility hardware, one an athlete in a boot and another with a cast and crutches. I joked that we all needed decorations for our metal, plastic, plaster, and Velcro. I told them I'd broken a foot bone years before the RA and had glued plastic sparkly jewels from a hobby shop up and down the metal supports.

After that class, I retreated to my office, sat, and leaned the cane against another chair. In the dark I relaxed my cheerful game face and let exhaustion surface. The cane's flower print glinted dimly in the gray snow-light filtering from the window. *Don't cry*, I told myself, *or your face will be a mess for the next class*. I inventoried the aches and stretched. I noticed the pain to ease my panic about it. *Don't pretend you're not in pain. It's just pain.* This wasn't the life or the body I wanted. Not only that, I wasn't a version of the self I knew—and so was I still me? I did not know whether I would ever be bipedal again. I felt a kind of clawing, a desperate urge to take hold of anything that reminded me of myself.

What reared up in my mind was a childlike hope for reclamation. Like my joke in class about the jeweled boot, I needed stickers for the cane. And I needed attention, any kind of response from the void, any "you-go-girl" available and a collective crowdsource project to make a container for this heaviness.

I opened a browser and typed into Facebook:

"I have a project and a trade for you. I have decided my cane needs decoration. Do you have any cool stickers? If you send me one, I will send you a surprise in return . . . I have decided this thing needs to be way more beautiful and sexy and fabulous than it is. It needs to be a presence, not an absence."

Even when healthy, I never would have described my body as conventionally beautiful, sexy, or fabulous. But this was Facebook lingo with its celebration of audacious female-ness among my friends and acquaintances, and I took it as a sort of fairy-tale act-as-if. In framing the cane for my friends, I was forced to implicitly describe myself in terms I would normally shrug off as too positive or celebratory. But yes—I suppose in some fashion I had a body that was unconventionally

wonderful, sexy, fabulous, or at least serviceable and strong and completely lovely, though its joints were now inflamed and beset. *My* joints.

And the cane also needed to become mine, or its blankness would
subsume me, and I would become also not-mine. I saw that I needed
silly stickers, a messy art project like my own sticker collection from
grade school, prized scratch-and-sniffs and glittery Lisa Frank dragons
on shiny wax paper, stored safely in a metal box decorated with hearts
in primary colors.

Children use stickers as a way to mark territory, to claim mass-
produced adult items like furniture and notebooks with the creatures
of the imagination, with stars and unicorns placed at odd angles with a
smatter of small hands at a child's eye level. A sticker collection was an
arsenal of childhood, ready to mark a corner of the world as claimed,
as still childhood, as unscary.

Within an hour, friends rushed to my office in the middle of their
serious academic days, one with a sheet of tiny, multicolored smileys
and another with an adhesive Arc de Triomphe. My friend Emily, who
brought the Paris stickers, knocked and leaned in. I ushered her in and
then surprised her by bursting into despondent tears. She shut the door
behind her and said, "Oh honey . . ." She wrote down the name of a
massage therapist. And if I hadn't asked for stickers, I wouldn't have
cried to her by accident and wouldn't have received that phone number.
The massage therapist wouldn't have helped me figure out how exactly
to soothe an inflamed ligament, which would return back to normal
functioning over the next two months.

In response to the Facebook post, friends near and far over the next
three weeks sent real envelopes with real adhesives inside. Some of these
friends I'd never even met in real life. I got sticky Frida Kahlos and
slogans from yo-yo companies, shiny jewels and political slogans. I got
a very large and crazy sticker, bigger than my entire head, for a puppet
museum in Germany. I got unicorns and bottles of wine and sheets of
glittery jewels. These envelopes showed up in my mailbox each day to

buoy me through the darkest time, the time when I thought disease was taking away my style and rendering me invisible even to myself.

In the previous year, I had read Anatole Broyard's *Intoxicated by My Illness,* which describes the noted critic's cancer—not as a battle, that clichéd image of war; just a coexistence that ends with all parties fading to not-being. At first I thought Broyard was being flip when I read that "every seriously ill person needs to develop a style for his illness." He described this as the antidote to "falling out of love with yourself." Later in a bout of pain, I realized this was an instruction manual, and I needed to take it seriously. I, who pulled on clothing as an afterthought, needed to seek out fabrics that soothed my skin, bright patterns and necklaces that made me smile, lest depression claim me. And I needed the cane to be the staff of strength on my side instead of against me.

To claim some space on the cane myself, I ordered a tiny bumper sticker, "This Machine Kills Fascists," the slogan that had graced Woody Guthrie's guitar. I stuck on a slogan for a muffler company called "Cherry Bomb," and someone gave me a sticker that said, "Art is not a thing—it is a way." There's a sticker from New Orleans and a Hello Kitty up near the handle. I put the Frida Kahlo one on in a hurry because I was so excited, and I kind of messed up, leaving a tab of sticker in the back that won't quite adhere to itself. I had to cut the slogan about art in order to fit it along the curve of the cane, but that one still has ripples in the surface. Overall, the effect is kind of a mess, and that is good. The collage is smattered and overlapped, a joyful explosion of adhesives that draws more attention and brings more joy than an anonymous metal pole.

People stop me now to admire the cane. They want to check out what is curved all over it. The pin that makes the height adjustable is covered by a sticker, but I won't be adjusting it anytime soon. To be honest, the cane really is mine. It's at the height I need, and that's that.

I won't pretend the cane is a triumph or that I love it. Or do I love it as a girl loves a stickered notebook or folder? I like it as a sign of my childishness in the adult world of functional implements. On some days the cane is now almost invisible to me, because it looks mottled and battered and sloganed and random like the rest of my life, which has allowed it to fade into the background. I suppose I do love it, now.

The cane itself seems happier when it folds away into hibernation; I know I'm projecting happiness onto it, but it is a version of my face and life looking back at me, one I admire. On days when I hate my disease, I don't have to also hate a simple object that keeps me upright. I have let myself understand that I can still mark this territory as mine.

I still have to do something about the lanyard. I have visions of weaving it with red embroidery thread, hanging beads or a shell from the end, but I don't want to get carried away. Or maybe I do.

INTERSTATE AND INTERBEING

Rubber tires strike the chord of asphalt on Interstate 95. The tone and overtone waver around B-flat to D, melding and separating like a Tuva throat-singer's moan in the mountains of Mongolia. The hum peaks feverishly at 7 a.m., whining into my window with the song of lateness and watch-checking and elsewhere. The strip of highway vibrates about two thousand feet from my ear as I lie in bed holding my glowing phone over my face. I scan work emails from disgruntled or confused students. I switch to Facebook and descend down into the blue column with pictures of apocalypse, dinner, and vacation, an escalator without end. The rushing is samsara, the Buddhist term for worldly suffering. I pull myself to sitting, my ass where my head has been, and set the timer on my phone for twenty-three minutes, an arbitrary chunk of time to meditate. I open my head and close my eyes. What comes in is the highway.

I live near this artery at the eastern edge of the United States, about an hour north of New York City. Our little house is jammed in the elbow of a curved road behind a Walmart built over a Superfund site we didn't know about when we bought the house. Our little, yellow house with blue shutters sits tightly alongside the other houses with their shoulders hunched around their aluminum-sided ears. In the early morning I am most aware I do not live in a big, quiet house in the pines.

Does Buddha love me less because I live near the highway?

Highways are a kind of *nirmanakaya*, part of the path, anything that helps humans fulfill their goals toward enlightenment. Without the highway we could not get to places that might wake us up. This spring I was sleepy, too busy, and exhausted from work to plant flowers outside. The perennials came up anyway, lilies and cornflowers that have taken over half the lawn in front of the little, yellow house with blue shutters.

Inside the house, ass on my pillow, timer running on my phone, surrounded by the whine of the highway, I am awash in the cycle of comparing and insecurity. The *heee* of the highway sings *what-if, what-if.* My first reaction when I greet my physical pain in the morning is "I don't want it." I want other things: I want a lot. I don't want this body. I want a different one. I don't want these sensations.

I imagine drawing close to that concrete vein two thousand feet away, each person in each metal carapace crossing an invisible laser line across the highway at the point closest to my house. I touch all the lives in all the cabs of trucks and cars passing at such high speeds, all sad and giddy and worried and dying. The worst day, the best day, and someone is unhappy with you right now, all fixed in this jelly of motion. All the rounded eyeballs and rounded skulls of the wrinkled children with their wanting course alongside me.

I go into the kitchen for another cup of coffee, and I hear the rush of tires in their midday song, trucks singing low and long notes of *om.* I touch all the lives in all the cabs of trucks and cars passing so close to me at such high speeds, all sad and giddy and worried and dying.

PAIN WOMAN TAKES YOUR KEYS

Writing delivers sheer absorption and physical confrontation with myself. I step into the cockpit, fueled by a beautiful morning bubble of caffeine. The glowing screen dares me and taunts me: Make something out of nothing. Make a sentence that sucks slightly less than what you see in front of you. Make it true, whatever true might me.

Writing has been a solace for most pain in my life, partly because of the focus it requires. The focus of writing leads me to a kind of trance, with the happy side effect of an almost-complete separation from this mortal coil. I forget my body and my surroundings. As I've lately confronted more physical chronic pain, the focus of writing often delivers an hour or two in which the aches in my bones are erased.

I've enjoyed this physical numbness, and there have been days when writing has been my only relief.

Then there are other days where I am simply not myself. Past that point I inhabit a strange, altered consciousness brought on by the pain. Over the past few years I began to worry that the fogginess and ache of autoimmune disease would destroy my writing. This would be a triple loss: shutting out something I do for my job, something I do for joy, and something I do for escape.

As I have done for years, I sit down every weekday morning and aim for my hour-plus at the computer screen. Some days there's nothing there, but I go to the page even when nothing feels promising, just for the relief of playing with words.

Some days in the last year, all I could make was a blog post. My writing voice on those days felt as if it had far less energy, less scope. It seemed obvious: I was not a writer but a woman who, in fact, could barely string sentences together. Writing with the submerged pain-voice feels like using a pinhole camera instead of a wide-angle lens.

Last year in such an altered pain state, I gave up on serious writing and wrote a blog post called "The Shadow Syllabus," kind of a fugue-state reflection on what I think about as an essayist and human while I write syllabi for my classes. I put the piece up on my blog and walked away from the computer, feeling defeated. This was all I could muster for the day, but I was practicing being kind to myself by doing a little and then stopping. To my shock, the post went viral, linked and shared by various educators around the world, cited and reblogged and so on. Then the next year when syllabi time rolled around, it started up again.

This has been wonderful but strange, because the Pain Woman who wrote that post doesn't feel like the woman I know who has been writing with my hands for twenty years, the woman who tries so hard to build essays with complex and multilayered sentences. Pain Woman has a different voice. She has a kind of messianic confidence that I do not have in my normal writing or even in my normal living, and this is the most shocking thing. The "me" I know or have inhabited most of my life is so ready to apologize for my point of view. I come at my writing sidelong, midwestern, nerd-female, postbullying, still gun-shy of ever saying something directly.

Pain Woman gives no shits. Pain Woman has stuff to tell you, and she has one minute to do so before she's too tired. Pain Woman knows things.

My non-pain voice searches for metaphors to entertain you. She aims to fascinate with far-reaching, pretty, solar-system lava curlicues, hiding behind constructions that might allow you to forget for a second that you are even looking at a woman at all.

Pain Woman takes your car keys and drives away.

This emergence of a distinct second voice brought on by my physical disability and medical issues raises several strange issues about writing. First, it confirms my long-held suspicion that the phrase "find your voice" is inaccurate and probably unhelpful. It implies that voice is a needle in a haystack—an elusive entity we have to catch and then put on. Actually we're swimming in our multiple voices, and all we have to do is listen to ourselves. This is tougher than a game of capture the flag, hard and painful. To hear our voices, we have to grapple with what we hear, which might be different from our idealized or hypercritical versions of ourselves. We all have multiple voices, I believe. What's strange is that, at least in my case, some of the voices remain completely submerged until other voices are sloughed away.

I'm mystified by the pain voice for reasons having to do with craft. If her writing is sometimes very powerful, as judged by reader responses to my blog posts, I wonder whether I have been trying too hard—or using the wrong muscles—with what I have known of my writing. My collection of voices includes Academia Woman, the Editorial/ Demonstration Pissed-Off Woman, Dreamy Essayist Fragment Girl, and Hayseed/Punk Rock Girl. Have I been trying too hard with all of them? Or have I not yet found the way to be direct, and only pain can strip away the artifice that hides me from myself on the page?

Or maybe I have had to learn writing first in order to unlearn it and strip it down to Pain Woman when she is required. Maybe my sentence weight-lifting lets me thread this needle of pain with a different voice when I need it.

This reminds me, too, that when I believe I am at my best as a writer, I may not be meeting my reader's needs. Sometimes when I think I'm humming along making beautiful sentences, I might just be doing a schtick I have honed over time, using one old routine when I could try others. Pain Woman's emergence and her strange rhythm, her simple plodding confidence, all make me wonder how each writer's voices develop and morph and ferment and merge over time.

Pain isn't making me a better person. It binds up my concentration, chops it into tiny pieces, thus requiring me to speak on the fly with thoughts made strange. This strange-making is often said to be the task of art: to cast the world in an unfamiliar light. Pain Woman is unable to access the routines and habits I've picked up, the automatic scripts, of what I see as my style. She can find the shadows and scraps of them, but she has to use them to make something else.

I don't know what I would have to say about any of this, but Pain Woman would say: You have more options than the writerly self you think you should be writing through. Take your own voice and destroy it. Shatter it and look at yourself in each of the glinting pieces.

IV

BITCHINESS AS TREATMENT PROTOCOL

ON GRATITUDE, AND OFF

I recently read a blog entry in which a woman with multiple sclerosis lists the ways she is grateful for her illness. The disease, she writes, has improved her life in concrete ways, giving her a purpose and a community of fellow sufferers.

I am both drawn in and repelled, reminded of the mysterious similar statements I've heard, the greeting card variety of spiritual transcendence—*I'm grateful for my cancer*. Then and now I cringe. More than that, however, I ache for those others with cancer who are not grateful, who hate the silent comparison they are thrown into, those who are just bitter about their cancer, who want to throttle it, who have been laid low by it.

I understand what this woman means, but I wish she would not have said it. Or maybe I don't want to delete her blog entry. What I want is more precision with the blunt language of gratitude. I want more separation from the implicit requirement that we be happy for everything that happens to us—that we not mourn as a part of being grateful. I want release from cartoon gratitude.

Transformation happens through suffering. I have been remade by difficult experiences that forced me to ask for help, that forced me into community, which has become a keystone of my life. But there's simple emotional algebra to parse, I suppose. If I am grateful for the transformation, for the community, am I thus required to go back to the root causes and also to be thankful for those elements? Each element is a part of the transformation, but the equivalence needs an algebraic function to change into its new form.

I feel a remarkable range of other things besides grateful. I feel resentful, envious, curious, cornered, and fearful. I feel a blank space that eludes language between me and the various illnesses that have touched my life and my body. There are so many silences. There is a gap. Lack of precision with language hides my deep anger at conditions beyond my control that have stolen relationships or that have marked me permanently and changed the course of my life.

And yet my grief emerges also because I felt entitled to a different story, because my imagination claimed other futures, because I wanted and got so much. I recognize that the gratitude story is real because it says and means, *How amazing that we get anything at all.* This is good spiritual guidance and terrible politics.

I am not grateful, I suppose, partially because I still have an alternate version of my life in my head: a version of me that continues on, free of these obstacles. She is blithe, less bitter, more well-traveled; she has a much better wardrobe and is never irritated. I wonder about her, that untouched woman, and I wish I were her. I see very clearly the ways in which I have been limited by illness as I compare myself to this fantasy woman. The path out of this fantasy-envy or spiritual unrest is acceptance, and I have that too.

I don't think I am grateful for the actual causes of my suffering— the addiction riddling my family tree and more recently rheumatoid arthritis. Instead of saying "thank you," I have often cried with my arms draped over the steering wheel or screamed in the echoing glass quiet of my car. I am in a complex relationship with those causes, an inextricable intimacy that does feel a lot like love. But is love the same as gratitude?

I can say I love my disease when I think about how close we are, how well I know it, and how much it has pushed me. I also love the complex web that addiction has pressed into my life. To me love is knowledge, is intimacy, is a closeness that is not always easy but usually challenging and rewarding. Whether one has been forced into such a relationship through luck of birth or genetics, "love" covers this web as a shorthand.

So that's something surprising: I love the causes of my suffering. But even this is not gratitude.

In a way, I love this space of illness because it is me—marked, imperfect, hollowed out by the weather that has beset my frail encampment on a cliff in an arid, stony place. I love this whole particularity because I have connected with others on a level I might not have thought possible otherwise. I love the particular hard and barren landscape on which I have made a home. I love my own ability to live here. I love others who live on similar landscapes in a particularly poignant way because I know the mingled collection of ache and triumph and resignation their lives must contain.

My world, as the result of these illnesses, has become incredibly subtle. Like an expert in any field, I find that the hours spent feeling and analyzing these syndromes have resulted in a complex knowledge of shades of emotion. I am much more self-aware than I might otherwise be. I have several other lenses through which to see life in general, and those alternate lenses have helped me in challenges that have nothing to do with the illnesses themselves.

So with regard to illness, I have love and even true acceptance—at times, in moments, as shifting as the clouds, to be replaced in the next half hour with fits of rage and black doom and envy. I have all of these things. But gratitude demands more from me than I am willing to give.

If I said I were grateful for these conditions, it would seem as though I were saying "I would choose this." Gratitude's twin definitions are "pleasing" and "thankful." To say "thank you" to the universe for the pain itself seems like a level of abjection that insults the dignity of the ill. Pain is real, after all—and it is only through appreciating the gravity of suffering that I have been able to see its real effects and, therefore, my real accomplishments in living with it. Not everything is "good." It is only in proclaiming something clearly bad—a life twisted with addiction, a hand gnarled by arthritis—that we have any yardstick for understanding the true negative impact these conditions have on a life and thus the accomplishment of abiding them.

I am glad I am surviving this in this way. I am glad that people got together to devise collective nets to catch and repurpose sorrow. Sorrow doesn't need us to be thankful for it.

The Christian notion of taking suffering personally is as a cross to bear. Was Jesus grateful for his cross? He asked, "Let this cup pass me by." We didn't even ask of Jesus himself that he say thank you. He didn't run away, but nobody forced him to smile.

In any serious loss, including illness, "grief is a normal and healthy experience," writes David Malham in the *New York Times*. "But so is resilience." To simply say one is grateful for cancer hides the massive grief that must have been experienced before the momentary proclamation of gratitude. The mourning and the response to mourning—resilience, that wellspring—make the meaning in illness. That is not illness itself creating its own solution; that is the human heart and mind.

The meaning contained in the illness experience is precisely *not* that I would choose it. The meaning is that it has chosen me, and I have adapted. This resilience—my own, very messy, and struggling resilience as revealed to me over the course of years—has awed me. But the seed of it is a bad seed. It is not a blessing. We cannot pretend, I believe, that everyone is living the life of the blessed. Suffering is real.

I doubt whether any deity asks an unenlightened being to say, "More, please." What we hear as God might be the shadow of America that asks us to smile and wave as our personal ships go down.

I should be happy for these people who can say they are grateful for hardship, that they have found a resting place. Maybe I am. They have achieved a state of peace with a difficult situation, a peace I can only imagine and envy.

I don't believe they are always in that state, though. I know the bubbles of peace, the moments of insight and transcendence that cause someone to go to the keyboard and proclaim. But those happy sentences hide all the hours of prosaic misery in a cloak of shame and, therefore, make those hours seem less honorable.

We chide each other: be aware, be grateful, be present every moment, as if gratitude were the virtue of the day. Gratitude is the privilege of those who can stop time. Grateful is a large, heavy, huge proclamation that steps out of the minutiae of the day. I cannot say I am grateful because I am so often subsumed by the day instead of mastering it, proclaiming my dominion over it or my emotional summary.

One recent morning I felt the nature of time as slippery, recoiling, eelish. The minutes slipped forward from 6:50 to 8:13, every moment's effort necessary to get myself and an eleven-year-old out the door with papers slipped in correct folders, insulin shot into the cat, two lines of liquid eyeliner, two pieces of salami on two pieces of buttered toast, 600 steps on the Fitbit, seven or eight spritzes of hairspray, two blurbs of toothpaste on two toothbrushes, four socks and four shoes, two book reports signed.

And all the while I floated above pain's substrate, shadowed by the blur of a night in which I chased sleep and moved from the bed to the couch. This morning I pushed through curtains of sadness. Now I am fatigue-blasted into a kind of wonder, incredulous at presence itself, that March 23 is a pinned butterfly, a tiny pivot. I am awed at each day I have survived and swum against the pounding surf of emails, requests, need to do, gummed envelopes with coupons to remit. How does anyone survive?

This, too, is not gratitude at my disease. This feels in shorthand like wonder about the disease, but it is actually awe at seeing up close the gaps in time's connective tissue, watching as the self emerges in a shadow blur despite being blasted into fragments.

Pain shatters time into a mosaic, and this is fascinating. I have been grateful to get this up-close view of the glinting tiles of each moment.

This is gratitude for the nature of time itself, not the disease.

I'm interested in the way an abstract emotional concept, like love or gratitude, can be stretched and turned into its opposite.

From inside one's soul, the word "grateful" is a blurred upwelling, a bounteous prayer.

From another person's lips, "I am grateful" can be an open space, a reminder to fill in that blank for one's self. Go back, examine your minutes, look for the ways in which time slows down, and the mosaic shines.

From above, "be grateful" can be a ladder down into shame. You can never be grateful enough, you ungrateful, selfish thing.

Because gratitude is real, it is also powerful as a weapon, a complex prayer turned to simple corporate pill. Pop-psychology and women's self-improvement magazines urge presence, awareness, and gratitude: *Savor it. Pay attention now before they're grown.* An autonomous impulse to reflect becomes a threat when it is turned into a commandment. *Be grateful you live in such peace and security.* (Fear the outside; they want what we have and will take it away). *Don't complain; be thankful.* (Just take what you get and be quiet.)

I refuse to be grateful for global warming merely because of the new way it has taught me to look at glaciers. Glaciers glint with blue-enough grandeur, cutting through time and rock, without the abbreviated, foreshortened life we have forced upon them.

Illness and suffering do create altered emotional states. Everyone who's had the flu recognizes that shining moment of getting up and feeling the first glimmers of health return. The orange juice: so tangy and orange. The clouds outside: resplendent. And I can theoretically see the argument that one might say "thank you" to the flu for delivering that moment, except for the fact that one can also arrive at it through many other routes that are less uncomfortable. Simply taking a nap or a run, having sex, talking with a friend, crashing one's car, being confronted with a financial challenge—these all change our viewpoints if we let them. So it is not the illness itself or its difficulty that is the crux of the perspective shift. The key is our changeability, the human mind's ability to reframe, reframe, reframe.

Sometimes when I'm sick and I actually admit that I'm being completely mowed down by illness, I have a momentary surge of gratitude for the release of acceptance itself. Illness has forced me to temporarily let myself off the hook. I can just be ill, and I must abandon what previously seemed essential—work tasks, cleaning, the next to-do. In this state, I see the things that I normally would ignore in my relentless quest to get stuff done. Specifically, I see that the urgency involved in completing a mundane task is a loss of perspective. It's not that big a deal; what's a bigger deal is the matter of my body's overwhelming signals of pain. This body needs rest. I collapse, and that feels delicious. Even the pain that I feel in those moments becomes a kind of friend, because I stop fighting it and begin to catalog it. I see that I can handle this twinge, that roar. It becomes less of a monolithic force.

Illness has forced me to let go. But this, too, is not a gift that illness brings. Like the wreckage unleashed by a typhoon, the destruction of illness is not equivalent to presents raining from the sky. The release that comes from illness is the effect of my own cognition in the face of the illness. There is a flame in humans—in the spirit, the soul, and in the body and between bodies—that sparks as a response to this lens-shift. I am profoundly grateful for that spark. I am grateful to be alive and to have a brain that makes meaning after meaning after meaning.

We want to make illness into a friend or an enemy. We want to tame it and give it a face. But its inscrutability, the awesome depth of its silence and its persistence and its unknowability, are its central characteristics. I have to honor the unknown and my own ability to contain this unknowability at the core of my life. I cannot be grateful for something I cannot contain, something I don't know the edges of, something whose future and past I don't understand. Illness is wild; it will devour us all. We can be at peace with that, but it is our minds and bodies that create the responses to it that make meaning, make sense, and make connection.

Then again, it could also be that this idea of gratitude repels me so because I know I have to reckon with it. Maybe this "grateful for my illness itself" is a destination marker on the horizon, a point of surrender in my future. It triggers deep fear: maybe I am not yet sick enough to be forced to curl up with my illness and thank it. Maybe there is a line one can cross, after which one's perspective is utterly changed, and one has then been completely claimed by illness, made *into* illness, speaking on behalf of illness itself. I resist this; I don't know whether I'll get there, but I don't want to get there. It probably isn't a matter of choice. But I understand that suffering is varied, and that any suffering can theoretically provoke a profoundly changed perspective.

I am not grateful for more acute suffering, which can also embitter and destroy. I don't want people to suffer, and I don't want to require them to welcome the destroyer itself. I want them to love themselves and all of their varied noble reactions in the face of destruction.

LIFE IS GOOD[1,2,3]

1. As if the gain itself, the good, the fat, were the point, as if loss weren't what tied us to other people and broke apart our fake shimmering shells, as if loss weren't the true wealth, the shape-shifter. As if this assertion of sunshine would be enough to blot out any depression—and much worse, as if one should, therefore, be ashamed to have the momentary flash of petulance: life *sucks*. As if teenage rebellion against life could be ignored out of existence with a smile. As if we could ever understand life—think of that—all of life, and declare it good, in the process stretching the word "good" out far enough to slacken it to the size of the universe; yes, let's make them equal, and then we will be safe, take the precision of a narrow field and put in an equal sign so that we don't have to worry anymore. As if you were also in complete union with the reverse insight, the Buddhist *om* of universal acceptance of all phenomena, enlightenment itself, a roiling hell of death confronted, not captioned with a smiley face. You wear this shirt when faced by cancer, squeezing out the drops of shimmering life from a cup of orange juice, and I get that part, I revere that attention to the particular in the face of the extreme, but isn't that said with a shiver, in a serious font, whispered among loved ones, and not slapped on a bumper sticker? Maybe a smaller type size, and not comic sans. Its goofy joy strikes me as gloating when it appears on your Jeep's spare tire,

facing me in traffic, or is it a kind of anti-intellectual smugness that claims space for simple joy, as if the simple things are the most true? In a way I get this is true, even when not stoned: Dude, cheese; air; teeth. But as if rejecting the complex were any way to live. As if it's almost on purpose that this slogan would stymie me, ease me into a world where overthinking is extinct. As if in nostalgia for a time that never existed, where things were imaginarily simple, where we might imagine we found union through gratitude toward every blessed blade of grass. And yes, I get that too, but secular gratitude also turns on itself, because the spiritual container is too weak, a water balloon, too much of a product, and it easily turns into a corporate appropriation, a shaming where we are required to say thank you, thank you to every boss and hellish moment, be grateful they gave you anything at all. As if any disruption in normal goodness were a lack of appreciation, as if orange juice were all we needed, as if.

2. This led me to obsess, to research the company (a pair of white, Boston brothers, wealthy now from selling T-shirts) and to follow the evolution of the company's slogans, the move after 2010 from poor design to an appropriation of seventies-style graphics, washed-out, never-been-there vintage and, of course, Namaste. They, too, sing America. As if I could relax into it for just a second, and then I would understand everything.

3. in a wind tunnel of fragility at the edge of the crumbling world.

DEAR NOTED FEMINIST SCHOLAR,

Thank you for your amazing enthusiasm regarding my writing, and for your wonderful book. Thank you for noting the overlap of the personal and the political and for your repeated discussion of embodiment in your scholarship. Thank you for the four emails in tones of increasing urgency asking me to come to a conference next fall to speak on a panel, and for the huge honor of viewing my work as important, and for giving me an opportunity that five years ago I could have only dreamed about. Thank you for not taking no for an answer, and for making me articulate exactly what it means to live with a disease that is both painful and energy sapping. Thank you for making me detail the obstacles, which include the fact that any lengthy travel in the middle of the semester will make me sick and thus destroy weeks of lucid work and family time, and that I already have one long trip for work blocked out for those months, and that I cannot do another without risking immune system collapse and weeks of pain. Thank you for your inability to understand—despite all the feminist celebrations of embodiment— that sometimes bodies create complications and limitations. Thank you for forcing me to explain and confront the fact that I live in a state of active mourning, which includes the absence of a shared way of knowing the world, and for reminding me about the invisible isolation of being at odds, at the edge, unusual. Thank you for subtly guilting me into pushing myself to attend this conference and for forcing me—after once giving a brief mention of my disease—to detail its implications for you, and for thus forcing me to rise from a vague, guilty, weepy sadness into a clear anger at your pursuit of your own agenda. Thank you for reminding me that the world of persona and star-creation is one that excludes bodies with illnesses and that social capital is created with bodily appearances attained only with multiple hours of sitting in cars and trains and planes in vats of bacteria and virus-laden air. Thank you for making it all crystal clear for me, sharp-edged, and for turning me toward anger instead of self-pity.

All the best,
Sonya

V

INTIMATE MOMENTS WITH THE THREE OF US

A PAIN-SEX ANTI-MANIFESTO

My husband and I sat in our car in the parking lot of a sushi restaurant in North Carolina, making notes on the chronology of our sex life. We had five days left of a lazy week at a beach rental with his family.

That morning, instead of writing, I had clicked over to Facebook and found a call for the "sex" issue of a high-profile women's magazine. I dashed off an email to the editor with a thumbnail sketch of my sex trouble. I didn't think I'd hear anything back, because our story doesn't have the redemptive arc of the happy ending.

My husband and I had enjoyed a year and a half of wild and crazy dating sex before I got sick with rheumatoid arthritis. Suddenly issues of endurance, certain positions, and even whether I could have sex on a certain day were all completely unreliable and nonnegotiable. I had taken my hips completely for granted. On days when I couldn't move them, I turned away from him in tears. Then we had to do something even more awkward than get naked and have sex. We had to *talk* about sex. Often. He was fine with it, but for me—feminist, writer, word-person—it was agony.

That night, the magazine editor replied with interest and sympathy, wanting more details. And then I was mortified. Byline avarice and ambition had made me throw my gauntlet down way beyond my comfort level.

I walked to the bedroom, where Cliff was sprawled on the bed reading a presidential biography.

"So this big magazine might want this article about our sex lives," I said.

My memoirish proclivities had now pushed my husband into the awful situation of potential public exhibitionism for the sake of my writing. I felt like a gambling addict having to come clean about a major loss, confessing the way I'd put the family in jeopardy. And this subject was so painful; why exactly did I want to expose the nerve—not to mention various other organs—to strangers?

He looked up from his book. "Cool!" he said. "That's great, babe." He was so awesome, and I was so (metaphorically) screwed. I moaned. The normal part of my personality—shy, if you can believe it, and a little bit of a vanilla-prude—was enraged at the "writer"/attention-whore/daredevil.

"Oh my God," I said. "It's *sex*. What was I thinking?"

We excused ourselves from the family to have a private dinner and talk-down.

"Just make a list," he said. He was right. I needed narrative. A timeline and bullet points would help make sense of it. "We had one idea when we were here two years ago."

I propped my notebook up on my thighs as he pulled into the sushi place. "That's right!" I said, remembering the low point during our last beach visit when we'd had a window of family-provided child care, giving us romantic time to sneak away. I'd been so wracked with pain that I slept through most of it.

I wrote down years in a list and struggled to fill in the blanks, asking him what year things started. He has a much better memory for the chronology; for me it was a big blur of negativity. We continued in muted voices in the sushi restaurant, leaning over the notebook page as we sketched the timeline of our devolution from dating sex to the "work-arounds" prompted by chronic pain. I focused on the list and on his gamely positive attitude to distract myself from my shame and dread. I'd never been completely confident about sex, though before chronic pain I considered myself okay at it—and now I was utterly remedial. I liked to be good at things, and I sucked at sex. Never mind that I had an "excuse"; I couldn't forgive myself for failing.

Although my joints had hurt for five years, the body part I'd had most trouble with was my brain. I felt inadequate, and then I felt inadequate for my inadequacy. The shame-spiral had pinned me to the bed at various near-sexy moments where my body wouldn't cooperate. I was in pain—which gave me a visceral and constant irritation toward my mortal coil. The state of being sick made me feel generally negative about myself as a sexy, functional being in the world, so I added a conceptual and emotional cloud of hate around the physical experience along with apocalyptic thinking about whether this evil would ever shift. *Then* when I tried to have sex and couldn't, I was angry very specifically at the body parts that were unable to perform, thus adding, for good measure, a third layer of body-hatred.

When I first got sick, I was determined to push myself to have "normal" sex as a matter of willpower. Gritting one's teeth and bearing it, however, does not lead to orgasmic relaxation. We waited for windows of pain-free time that also happened to align with child-free moments, and these seemed to happen as rarely as a lunar eclipse. We then moved to Connecticut so that I could start a new job, and I spent so much energy on my work life that I bottomed out physically. Stress amplified my pain, and sex was bad because it forced me to temporarily stop ignoring all of my flared nerve endings. My solution was not to make any kind of eye contact with my husband, which I hoped would make the whole issue of sex disappear.

This avoidance is hell on a marriage, and it couldn't last. My husband broached the subject, and we began going to a counselor to really talk about sex. I ended up crying a lot, not because I was sad but because I was so mortified that we were talking about a problem that I had somehow caused. On one level my agony and embarrassment shocked me, as I had considered myself a liberated and open-minded person. The truth was that I was open-minded about other people's lives, but not about my own. I was so angry I had to have sex at all when my body hurt. I was angry about the whole situation, angry I couldn't perform, and horrified that I had to list positions that hurt, sitting in a room with my husband and a therapist, all three of us fully clothed. It felt like the least fun threesome ever.

Counseling visits and awkward homework assignments ("Look deeply into each other's eyes . . . .") didn't magically solve things, but we began to have an evolving negotiation about what counted as "sex." We began to at least talk about it, and I got better at those conversations. After awhile, only about one in ten sex attempts would send me into a spiral of crying and self-loathing.

Let me not pretend, though, that I was remade as a Zen sexual being. I had another way to quantify my sex success and reduce my anxiety. I began to focus on making sex "count." I would aim to have good— "normal," "to completion"—sex, and that would keep things healthy in my relationship. After such a romp, I often felt like dying from fatigue and pain. But it was a worthy sacrifice.

This meant, however, that I developed an imaginary scorecard as a sex martyr. If I were going to walk a bed of hot coals through the inevitable pain, I wanted a point in the "win" column—and I defined "win" as a male orgasm, a very retro idea that would lead to him being satisfied and, therefore, being happy with me, and having the desire/problem sort of controlled for a while. This all sounds super-fun, right? Often I still had to stop partway through, moaning that I had failed, wasting one of our rare child-free/not-agony sexual lunar eclipses.

Eventually, we lay next to each other and began to talk about our personal sex-apocalypse.

My husband, still trying to reassure me, told me that anytime we could get naked and lie around together was a "win." I thought that was a nice idea and agreed to think about it as long as I could secretly hold onto my insecurities and worries about sex. This idea also did help with my hang-ups, and usually after relaxing with him for a little bit, I was able to have even a little bit of "real" sex, or to focus less on the end zone. He has continued to reassure me so often that I'm sometimes (like maybe 40 percent?) able to give myself full credit for a partial attempt and to remember that he still finds me attractive, because he constantly reminds me.

But back to the little article I had submitted. An edited version appeared in my email inbox with what I recognized as a standard closure in "magazine voice." I'd written these closures many times myself, an easy ending sentence to tie up messy life experience with the implication that things were simply super.

I mulled this over, realizing that once again I was back to the strange world of qualifying and quantifying sex, which I had tried so hard to ignore. I realized that, even while I wanted to be an easy writer to work with, okaying this change would be a complete lie in terms of my real life. I couldn't say our "sex life" was great. (The phrase "sex life" always weirds me out anyway, like it's another existence entirely, too close to "sea life.") I edited the last line to read that while our relationship is getting better and better, our sex life "works."

It's not "better." I'm not living the dream. It is sort of better than it was, but I'm still sick. As the Magic Eight Ball would say, "Ask again later."

Under normal circumstances my husband and I might not have needed to talk extensively about what works for us sexually and what helps us feel connected, but this situation has forced us to have those conversations. I think this has definitely brought us closer, though it has not been easy. It's made me mindful that I can't shut down physically, and that we have to have physical affection when we see each other even if it's not sex, which helps us both. Instead of wincing I hug him and tell him how cute he is—even when I feel like crap. And touching my husband doesn't always have to lead to sex, but if it does, I feel more comfortable these days giving up and calling it a good effort. Most days I still have a screaming third of my brain that sirens out: "FAILURE!" Sometimes my pain level is not so bad, our schedules align, and we're able to have a more abbreviated version of very good inventive sex with no pressure.

Whatever, though—who's counting? Only me, and the entire culture I'm soaking in. Sex is annoying when you keep score. We are supposed to worship sex as a wonderful egalitarian playland, which I realize is territory hard-fought for by sex-positive, second- and third-wave feminists. But I didn't feel liberated in the bedroom even before I got sick. I'm fraught, repressed, baggaged—and I'm okay with nudging myself forward with baby steps.

One of the unintended side effects of coming of age in the sex-positive, must-have-dildo era of the 1990s was an additional layer of shame that I wasn't where my peers claimed to be in terms of lube and glitter and orgies and whatever else they said was cool. Instead of feeling free to explore, I felt ashamed for the repression I carried around that made me regressive.

It wasn't that I didn't like sex. I did. And I had sex, and I was adventurous. But I was tetchy about it, weird. I sort of got through that and then was pulled backward by a series of personal mishaps in relationships that led to additional scars. So adding a chronic illness to the mix meant that when you take my clothes off and put me in a bedroom, I am much *less* comfortable than when I am fully clothed and talking with you over a cup of coffee. Sex might be natural for some people, but it's not to me. And that is not tragic, and I have only slowly realized that that is not something I need to immediately fix or feel embarrassed or ashamed about.

If sexualities were cars, mine would be a rusted-out, 1974 El Camino: weird-looking, and maybe the electrical system's a little shot, but it still gets me where I need to go at least part of the time, and I love it because it's mine. As they say, it has character, and the character is mine.

When I confessed to a friend that I thought sex was 75 percent annoying, she wisely replied, "It's fraught."

It's fraught. I'm liberated enough and free enough and let-it-all-hang-out enough to say: it's fraught, and it's gotten more fraught. And if I can't say that, I won't be able to claim any of my real experience, and if I can't admit what I really, really am, sex is out of the question as a real experience. I won't ever be sex-positive unless I can admit that sex-negative is where I'm at, and that's okay. The arc of having made peace with it, morphing into a character on *Sex and the City*—it's just not true. I'm not into finishing, happy endings, pressure of mutual orgasms, or tying it all up with a bow.

Sex will never be my friend again—and I'm getting to the point where that is *not a problem*. This is not a sin, though it feels like a sin to admit this in our sex-obsessed yet very conformist culture.

I still look at my husband and want to jump his bones. But these days I would need a ramp and an elaborate harness and pulley system as well as a good opiate to actually jump onto his skeleton.

I think lots of things are sexy. I think lots of things are beautiful and delicious. I admire bodies and senses and people. I very much enjoy being told by my husband that I look sexy.

Not being able to have sex the way I once did means that I have to stop idealizing the kind of sex you all say you have. It's not for me, and I'm actually not interested. I have quiet, intense sex, based on microns and millimeters, and I have it infrequently. Sex is art, not science. Sex is mystery, not football statistics.

To be honest, I still have to plan to feel like hell the day after we have sex, but whatever. I feel like hell anyway, so I'm getting better at feeling like hell.

For two talkers desperately in love, communication about sex has become more intimate than getting naked. It's not easy. In the past, I have loved men with whom I could never have opened my mouth and my heart like this. Pain pushed us to this point, and talking has sewn up the ways of loving each other that pain ripped apart. And love—active, continuous, searching, building—is sexy.

THE JOY OF NOT COOKING

I dumped a cold glob of Seafood Portofino—the remains of the previous night's dinner—into a bowl to microwave, unaware that I was approaching a deeply erotic moment.

"I could cook this summer," I said to my husband, who was making a salad for lunch. My husband's the food guy. He's a great cook, had made this fantastic meal the night before, as he did most nights—and I felt guilty. I tried to rally my limited enthusiasm and make it a project: Sonya Back in the Kitchen with Ingredients and Implements.

He chopped lettuce. "Why bother?" he asked.

I looked over at him. "Really?"

"Yeah. You do so much other stuff," he said, listing the tasks I tended toward: the bills, the insurance, the house stuff, the juggling of a full-time job plus overtime, the appointments, taxes, supplies for care and upkeep of the child, and so on.

The microwave dinged, and I looked at him and laughed the laugh of a lottery winner. I don't like to brag, but in this case it's clear I had received a windfall that had nothing to do with me. My husband is a very sexy man. Not just because of this, but this doesn't hurt.

Food and I get along fine, but we have a very casual-Friday relationship. I've been happy with the easy and low-budget combinations: a can of corned beef hash and a can of olives. A salad and a baked potato with some Indian lime relish. Hummus, after I made its acquaintance in college. Sandwiches. Mac and cheese with frozen peas thrown in. Scrambled eggs with ketchup. Cereal is fine for Seinfeld, but a woman who cooks like this is clearly a Communist.

I suspect that if I were a man, this would be "cute" or "normal," but there's always an uncomfortable pause when I make my confession. Questions are raised about what went wrong: upbringing, women in the kitchen, or maybe a horrible accident with a food processor?

Well, I did help start a grease fire while attempting to fry dough-nuts in a saucepan at a childhood friend's house. Although the ceiling and her eyebrows caught on fire, this was not the start of the cooking impasse.

Nor is it my mom's fault: she's a kitchen dynamo, filling the house with the scent of fried potatoes, pork chops, brats, and other German bedrocks. And she's open-minded and versatile. Our traditional family dinner on Christmas Eve was taco salad. (Yes, I am midwestern—but Bobby Flay. See, I know that name. I heard it from my sister.)

I existed fine with my handfuls of nuts and my grazing routines until I began my decades of cohabitation with various boyfriends. I noticed that my stomach would start to churn as the sun descended, and the evening was always hungry. My stomach wasn't rumbling; this was gendered five o'clock guilt. In the midst of writing, studying, doing full-time employment things, I always seemed to push away the thoughts of meal-planning until around four, at which point the only thing to be done was to make a salad or buy a preroasted chicken from the deli case.

No man I lived with ever looked at his watch, then at the significantly empty table, while tapping his foot impatiently. Maybe a few comments were made when it became clear no home-roasted chickens would appear from the oven. More than the lack of roast chickens, I felt a moral kind of failing: I should *want* to roast chickens, shouldn't I? The men I lived with often cooked lovely pasta dishes or used Crock-Pots with aplomb, and I like to think that I helped clear the way for this exploration into their inner Julia Childs.

Still, as I chewed their creations and praised them effusively, I resented the fact that they got extra credit for what I was supposed to do, for what I, therefore, did only grudgingly. To contribute to my own kitchen-shaming, I kept in my head an elaborate grade book of my food fuckups. This doesn't make me a bad kitchen feminist, of course—it means I'm having a little delayed ability to throw off our millennia of being chained to the hearth. Being pro-choice about cooking means accepting that some women just don't swing that way.

Around me, the kitchen memoirs began to appear. The Food Network's cooking shows listed every possible niche market, and a few times I watched—Bam!—waiting to be inspired by osmosis. But I always flipped back to CNN, mourning every evening when my inadequacy would be revealed between five and around six-thirty.

Was I lazy? No, I could work like a maniac. Was it possible to have a cooking disorder? I did have a uterus, and yet it didn't seem too talented at whipping up ganache. Why did I have this horrible Betty Crocker anxiety? I was bad at cooking, and taking the time to get better, while being observed by someone else whose dinner you would also ruin, was such a public way to fail. My cheapness didn't help; any ingredient off the beaten path seemed expensive and wasteful (because my inner landscape is the Spam-clad Midwest of the 1970s), and I don't like moving out of my comfort zone for some expensive ingredient or piece of kitchen implement that then demands to be continually employed. Also, I had this 1950s fear (an era I did not live in) that if I started cooking I'd wind up in the *Valley of the Dolls* with an apron tied around a 12-inch waist (which happened to no one I know).

Maybe I could blame a school musical from fourth grade, a sort of dystopian Martians-invade-and-everyone-sings-and-becomes-friends production. My job was to wear green face paint and stand very smartly in a row of my fellow Martians singing this song: "Energy pill. Energy pill. Never a favor or never a thrill! Fortunate is how we feel, as you can plainly see! We never worry for our next meal. It's always gonna be . . . an . . . energy pill. Energy pill."

I guess that vision of no food was supposed to be scary, but it sounded great to me.

Friends have tried to woo me to their side of the kitchen, thinking that if I just had a good experience, I'd be converted. I've cooked many lovely things, apple pies will boost any fledgling cook's self-esteem, and I do nice stuffed cabbage, a passable lemon-chicken thing, and I've sort of always liked ruining stir-fry. I have my private victories, and I have fed others well. I like wilted spinach with bacon and walnuts. I love food, but other people love it more.

I should just ignore foodies as I ignore football, because both cultures have nothing to do with me—but the culture of saffron and crème fraîche gets under my skin. The competitiveness makes me feel insecure, and this weakness is the insecurity of a woman who can't quite believe that domestic goddessery is really not expected of her. (Right?)

The posting of dinner pictures on Facebook puts me off a bit, but I have to tell myself these victorious images are meant for other audiences, not to shame me into getting back into the kitchen. Other people's dinners are not trying to make me feel inadequate.

During a recent fit of food pique, I sat down after cooking something less than lovely and googled "I hate to cook," hoping for a mommy online support group. Instead, I got the *I Hate to Cook Book* cookbook.

When I met the man who would become my second husband, I wooed him with egg sandwiches for lunch because that's the fixings I had in the fridge. I invited him over for dinners composed around the central axis of kielbasa combined with whatever was in the CSA box. Then I invited him over for dinner and handed him some meat when he walked in the door. I was a single mother raising a four-year-old and working full time, so he was very understanding. And because he liked food, he would rather cook something he enjoyed than eat something infused with my hatred and burned to a crisp because I was trying to read or write while cooking.

Then, once I had a captive cook in the house, my body—which subsisted so nicely on the ingredients I gave it—slyly collapsed. I began to develop a thyroid condition that everyone in my family seems to get, and then I got rheumatoid arthritis. No, I don't think the lack of saffron in my diet or absence of Le Creuset cookware had anything to do with my conditions.

Slowly over the past five years, in addition to taking my meds, I've been investigating the food component of autoimmune disorders. I started eating more walnuts. After taking on the initial challenge of a gluten-free diet, I began to see a slight decrease in my pain levels, and the added bonus was that fewer ingredient choices meant fewer things to attempt to cook. The truth is that I don't even care. I like making my own hideously colored green smoothies, which are the energy pill all Martians dream of.

KIDNEY STONE IN MY SHOE

One summer I decided to read the *Essais* by Michel de Montaigne, a Frenchman from the sixteenth century who is said to have invented the essay. I think I gave myself this task partly because of a lingering imposter complex about my surprising role as an English professor. As I made it past the 1,300-page mark, I was glad to get to this sentence: "I am not excessively fond either of salads or fruits, except melons. My father hated all sorts of sauces; I love them all." I sighed with relief when Montaigne stopped quoting Seneca and turned toward his real body, even when he dished about the details of his agony with kidney stones. Give me melons, give me sauces—just give me something specific, something with taste and smell and heft.

I had already been told that Montaigne taught himself to write as he wrote, developing his skill over time; nobody explicitly told me to avoid two-thirds of his work, but I should have. I didn't hear, however, that Montaigne's decaying body was also his writing teacher. As he ages and becomes ill, he becomes vulnerable and specific. Melons and kidney stones give me something personal, something that reminds me of Montaigne as a corporeal being. Montaigne's kidney stones bring him back to himself and make him strangely most alive.

Don't get me wrong: He's very approachable for the sixteenth century. He likes the simple life and the ordinary man, despite the fact that such pronouncements from a man of noble birth living on an estate sound at times like self-congratulation. Slogging through his statements about bravery and generals and military campaigns, I learned about Montaigne's preference for quiet, competent servants and his dislike of women who want sex too often. He's got a healthy self-regard that reads like a rapper's list of metaphors for greatness but without the rhythm: "Never was a man less inquisitive or less prying into other men's affairs than I."

The essayist's voice is often propelled by a sense of entitlement—the ability to pronounce a truth for the human race—which is a voice that many women have to struggle to attain. The memoir is easier; we say what has happened to us. That we know. We ask ourselves as we write whether we can say anything of universal relevance at all. Reading Montaigne let me understand that the voice of authority is part of the essay's legacy, and let me see that this is where I and many of my students and essays from minority viewpoints have struggled. We have struggled to create essays that "sound" like essays because we didn't have the entitlement to proclaim or the life experience that would lead us to assume people would listen.

It could be that I was primed to find fault with Montaigne. I had been told he was my literary father, as he is described as the originator of the essay and the art of digression. Literary nonfiction is continually trying to establish itself in academia as a serious form, and the essay and the name "Montaigne" are often used as shorthand for claiming our roots as a real field. In the end, it's not Montaigne that I object to, but the focus on him as the father of my genre, which makes me inevitably think of my mother and who she might be. This is especially painful in a field where so many female authors are not given their due as founders and guideposts, from Margery Kempe through to Annie Dillard and beyond. I would rather have eight sets of great-grandparents, male and female, than to be told I am descended from one man. As Montaigne would say, "They make me hate things that are likely, when they would impose them upon me as infallible."

Montaigne is also popular these days because he's avowedly secular; despite his statements of belief in Christianity, he blames none of his afflictions or his privileges on the power and judgment of an angry God. He despises cruelty and the wastes of war. He is open, questioning, and wandering—and in the end completely self-contradictory. However, he's not the only ancestor of nonfiction. I am partial to the sins and confessions of St. Augustine; what I love about that fourth-century work is what I also enjoy about many women authors: the focus on the body, the corporeal, the secret truths of physicality, and the inevitable complexity this introduces. While proclamation has been my weak point, I have always understood that an observation rings true when it is anchored in the detail of my life.

That brings me back to Montaigne's kidney stones, a painful affliction he focuses on for the last third of *Essais*. I don't enjoy his pain. It's just that his writing suddenly zooms into focus when he has a specific ailment, which forces him to tell me how he personally deals with pain. He writes about how his "pains strangely deaden" his appetite, and how his mysterious fits bring him a "crafty humility" because he can't know the cause of kidney stones or the timing of his attacks.

When he mentions his body, he is speaking to me as another human; I also have a crafty and painful condition, rheumatoid arthritis. He writes about his fear of death and his view of treatments and experience of pain itself with a thoughtful specificity that challenges me to do the same. I have feared that the focus on the body would sideline me as self-centered and narrow, a tag more easily attributed to female writers of nonfiction. When we write about the body, we are seen as writing for women—and not all women, but just those who share our specific condition; when men write about the body, they are seen to explore universals and write for humanity.

Montaigne's kidney stones are his path to humble brilliance through the vulnerability of describing illness. He burrows deep into the strange ease that happens after a fit of pain has passed, and I am there with him as a real presence. When he describes the way an illness strangely causes him to "think myself no longer worth my own care," I connect with the depression that pain brings on. He admits that death is easy to deal with as an abstraction, but the details of it bring him to tears. And he writes about the strange pain of bouts of wellness: "If health itself, sweet as it is, returns to me by fits, 'tis rather to give me cause of regret than possession of it; I have no place left to keep it in."

So I will go ahead and swagger, because the entitlement of the essayist's voice is a costume that Montaigne offers as a model. With my swagger, I will claim that the best writing of Montaigne deals with mortality and the body, and what Montaigne offers there is the willingness to switch moods, to describe things as they are, including the piss and the vomit. And not to be ashamed. Montaigne, as a man of wealth and noble birth, had a life that predisposed him to think that his offerings were worthy. But we can swagger like Montaigne, and I can try to write about my swollen knuckles without ever apologizing for being "depressing." Montaigne did not give a shit about that, and neither should we.

IF WOMAN IS FIVE

A few years ago, I walked into the grade-school cafeteria to collect my son from the YMCA after-school program. An older woman behind the desk asked me to wait while she checked through a pile of enrollment forms. Her fingers were gnarled at the joints and thickened at the fingertips, and the structure of the fingers had gone rigid and wavy. She flipped with some difficulty through the pages in the stack. My throat clogged with an impatience I tried to hide. I judged her as not too bright, maybe of a slow cognitive processing speed, as her finger pads struggled to arch and flick from one corner to the next.

The awfulness of my varied assumptions slipped into the spotlight of my awareness; it happens, these mental correctives against one's beastish nature. I saw myself linking intelligence to the working condition of fingers, maybe stemming from my own unconscious obsession with work and speed as a measure of one's value, a cruel equation for myself and others.

Then all thought stopped. The woman's knuckles loomed larger as I watched, as if those distended pockets of bone had become moons. Those slow knuckles and rippled fingers had been ravaged by advanced rheumatoid arthritis, my own disease, my possible future.

The blunted splay of a rheumatoid hand is a misconjugated verb, as if the articulate word of the hand has been misspelled. I admire hands, those creeping starfish, with a secret delight: a fancy manicure, a laborer's breadth of palm, the blur of a guitarist's solo. I began to be vain about my own hands in college, when I realized I would never be beautiful and looked beyond the win-or-lose binary of high school, hot or not. I could love my hands with their knobby strength, their uncomplaining service, and their automatic motions.

I use my hands when I talk, especially when I teach. Elbows splayed and sternum stretched, I scoop pockets of air, relying when my tongue fails on a pantomime of finger-drawn, imaginary diagrams. I think with my hands. If my hands were frozen, it might seem as though my speech itself were truncated. And if we think not with our brains but with our whole bodies' muscle memory, what blunted thoughts straggle from a world met with finger pads that refuse to alight where they are sent?

Prejudice against disabled people includes, among the spectrum of discrimination, a gut-level assumption that physical ability equals personality and cognition. That was my prejudice as I watched the woman's hands. I lumped her physical being with her ability to think and merged those two categories with her personality. Blurred, then dismissed.

When my son points out someone with a cane or a prosthetic arm in the grocery store, I gently chide, "There's nothing wrong with him. He was just born different. We're all different in our own way." I pretend I'm some sort of enlightened preschool teacher, as if all adults had arrived at this conclusion after a brief conference call.

Later when my son is bullied in school, I tell him that I was a bully in sixth grade. In the small bubble of that classroom, I was popular for the last time. I curled my hair in the crisp waves required in the early 1980s. I was friends with the cheerleader girls, who were considered beautiful. I got invited to their birthday parties, and in my joy at living what I thought was the perfect life, I leapt into a cruelty of confidence. We stood in line at the double glass doors waiting to go in from recess. We took a break from singing Queen's "We Will Rock You" to mock a girl named Renee. I believe now that she had moderate cerebral palsy, with thin legs and slanted hips. She shuffle-walked slowly, and her jaw was slightly tilted. We taunted her. I can't remember whether I ever started the taunts, but I remember the specific line of cruelty being that she was *mean* or *stuck-up* or some other vague dig at her character. We knew not to say "Ha ha, you can't walk like us," but we used the gut-level fear of something different, something wrong to put as much distance as possible between her and us—and to assert our supposed superiority, to show each other our daring and our devotion to the stupid ideals of beauty.

I tell my son that I still think about Renee and regret being a sixth-grade demon. I tell him that when you're mean to someone, it stays with you for the rest of your life.

Renee told us we were being mean and that we didn't have any right to talk like that to her. Her voice was high-pitched and clear, delivering sentences of reasoned response that showed she must have had a kind, supportive parent at home. She had been walked through the parries to being taunted. The teasing doled out from kids like us must have made her cry. I seem to remember her eyes filling with tears. The parent who heard those reports secondhand must have wanted to murder us all.

Renee had an ally, Mrs. Peterson, an older woman with blond, curly hair and blue eyeshadow, who was the teacher's helper in the classroom. Mrs. Peterson didn't like me because she knew I was one of the taunters, and she would stop us when she saw or heard the tension between the mean girls and Renee to set us straight, to embarrass us.

Mrs. Peterson didn't walk right either. She had a slight shuffle, but her limbs weren't thin and spindly like Renee's. Instead, her hands were twisted and scrunched and her elbows seemed frozen. She still managed to do classroom tasks, collating and stapling, delivering handouts, but she seemed to use her fingers as a wad, like flippers. When she stopped us, we knew that her ire came partially from the fact that she and Renee were of a kind.

But what was wrong with her? Could it happen to us? We didn't know; no one said. It turns out what happened to her could happen to us, is happening to me.

On a fall day in the park I walked beneath gum trees, their bare, mottled trunks lit golden, their fingerlike branches twisted like hands, each frozen in a unique shape, turned by layers of wind and days. The trees remind me of my Aunt Marie, who left the convent in Arkansas to find marriage. As rheumatoid disease crippled her, it was as if a sky devil had grasped her hands and limbs in a slow tornado and torqued. She went back to the convent, disabled and needing help with daily tasks, and she died in great pain.

The trees remind me of my mother's hands, which after years of aching are now rippling like the hard-packed sand near the shore when the tide goes out. The doctors told her in the 1980s that she had a kind of noninvasive rheumatoid arthritis that wouldn't cause disfigurement, yet she is changed. They told her to take lots of aspirin, and she has, for thirty-five years.

On a visit home recently I stared at her hands, then tried not to stare. I have always been in love with my mother's hands. She could do anything, my mother who has the strength of a German bulldog. She would laugh and flip someone the bird as they made fun of her. She would pad scoops of red ground beef into meatballs and patties. She would grab a coffee cup, make sandwiches, collect dishes, grab the phone, light a cigarette—all with her intelligent hands. She wore a gold ring with a red coral stone. She can hardly wear rings anymore.

My distaste at the disfigurement is grief. The hands I loved will never again be seen on this earth. My mother is alive, but a part of her is not as I remember. My distaste is also grief at my own transformation. I might pretend it is beautiful, end this with a reference to the tree's branches shining in the golden evening light, but that would be a lie.

Instead of a golden image regarded as a Wordsworth in repose, I will do violence but set out with purpose. I will use these hands exactly where they hurt and clench my knuckles until tears spring in my own eyes. I want to go back and rip out the roots of all of my assumptions. I want to debone and fillet my life like a fish, taking out the links between form and beauty, form and personality, form and being. The well-formed limb, the athlete, the enjoyment of the fine, the David, the Venus. I want to rip out my own disgust for the wretched, the twisted, the crumpled, the endings and leavings of bodies. I realize only that every single thing must be remade.

I will begin again, backward. I will start a new life from my own hands at this late and sorry date at the beginning of disfigurement. My fingers have begun to splay outward. They swell, and individual fingers twist in asymmetrical directions. I discard rings. I am on good, strong drugs, the privilege of this era and insurance and social class; I might be saved the rippling. But I see its early markers.

A mother gives birth, and then after a baby emerges, she wants to know: ten fingers? ten toes? A simple bit of math, and she believes this is the sign that all is well.

I have five fingers on a hand, and the family I came from had five members: mom, dad, brother, sister, me. I remember listening to Frank Black, the lead singer of Pixies, wonder aloud in "Monkey Gone to Heaven": "If man is five, then the devil is six . . ." His voice escalates to a high roar: "And if the devil is six then *God* is *seven*!"

If woman is five, she can take care of herself. She can lift a child, load a pickup truck, grab her keys, work, buy food. If woman is five, there is always freedom.

I think about all the ways I cannot serve others if my hands do not work: the elemental kneading bread, the cooking I do simply and not well, the image of a woman's hands hanging a sheet on a line, the patting of a child's warm forehead.

I can still do some of these things, sometimes, though the timing is not up to me. I can usually pour myself a cup of coffee, carry it downstairs, and I can type. I have not yet run up against a day in which all three of these are denied me.

Yet I am fighting my own simple math, my own outrageous assumptions about what qualifies one as functional. I discard myself, which means I have discarded others. I dismiss myself as less than human when the five rebel.

There is a movie with Juliette Binoche called *Words and Pictures* in which Binoche plays a painter who adapts to her limitations with rheumatoid arthritis. She lies on an office chair to hover over the floor and paint on a canvas, her hands in splints. I learn these details from reviews about the movie. I have not watched the movie. I should. I can't make myself. Yet.

Similarly, I declined to go to the exhibit of Henry Matisse cutouts at the Museum of Modern Art, though the art was on display for five months last year. These iconic images in bright colors were his last work, and I've always loved them, the blocky flowers and blue figures of women. With the help of assistants, he painted gouache color onto white paper shapes and tacked them up, covering walls in patterns, a vibrant breakthrough in his work necessitated by disability. The MoMA website does not mention disability as the source of his innovation, and I am wrestling with whether this is the best or the worst thing. Matisse used a wheelchair after surgery for cancer in 1941, which was why he turned to and pioneered the cutout method.

Matisse wrote, "Every day that dawns is a gift to me and I take it in that way. I accept it gratefully without looking beyond it. I completely forget my physical suffering and all the unpleasantness of my present condition and I think only of the joy of seeing the sun rise once more and being able to work a little bit."

I missed seeing these works of vivid color—even though I love Matisse, and I am a visual person and feed on color—because I was afraid. I was afraid because I thought the exhibit would somehow be sad instead of a temporary church to boldness. I rarely go into the city because it exhausts me, but I considered going because I knew this exhibit had something huge to teach me. And then I declined to learn it.

As penance or to hope I will be stronger later, I order a book of the cutouts online.

On a Saturday this past August, my husband and I visited a massive used bookstore I'd wanted to visit with him. On the way, we listened to a mix CD made for a friend's 50th birthday, and I danced in my seat to "Brick House" by the Commodores, funking it up as we coasted on the arched concrete past New Haven, and he shook with laughter as he drove. We found the rambling New England building and wandered amid the stacks. We gathered bags of books we'd always wanted to own. I carried one bag but then left it on a stool as I browsed, knowing wordlessly that he would come behind me and grab it, because he knows my hands.

After we paid, we ate scallops at a restaurant as the day grew overcast; we'd brought bathing suits but decided against finding a beach because my body was suffused with a dull, hot ache that meant I should avoid more exertion unless I wanted to risk a flare, a sort of immunological kickback. I don't know how these flares work; I strain for metaphors, but I know that it has something to do with exhaustion. Is it like stirring sediment in a bottle of pond water, or like waking tiny sleeping beasts? I know only this: sometimes I'm on one side of a line, and I know exertion would loosen and lubricate the achy joints. I have windows of freedom, and I dash through them like a child laughing. I push, clean, walk, and good air fills my lungs and pink fills my cheeks, and I am inhabited by the strong capable self I have always identified as "me." And then other times I am on the far side of that line, and I have to drop on the couch and hide.

The tired ache was creeping inside me as we ate, and on the drive home I played a game on my phone, a mind-numbing little dot-connecting thing I would have scoffed at in years past as a waste of one's attention and minutes. But now the object is to waste minutes, to be numbed, to get through, to be gone. And I like the colored dot game.

We parked in front of our yellow house, and I looked down at the mess I had to pick up on the floor of the car: a dirty travel coffee mug, my purse, a baseball hat. I opened the door and swung my feet to make contact with the driveway. Orange daylilies throbbed with late summer persistence as I passed the front of the van, scooping my keys from my purse. My husband unloaded the two plastic bags of books from the back of the van: the carrier, the helper, laden. My job was simple but I knew—no, I cannot ever know, I only cast backward into the previous minutes an understanding to paint the shock as less of a shock—that there would be trouble.

I didn't know there would be this much trouble, but it was simple. I put the key in the lock, and I could not turn it. Sometimes when they are bad, I make my aching flipper hands work with a sort of muscled nudge of bone and vectored force, but that was the first day I could not let us into the house. Not because it hurt but because I could not make my body turn the key.

I turned and left the step, went into the yard. My husband put down the bag of books and turned the key, opened the white door into the yawning darkness.

A DAY IN THE GRAMMAR OF DISEASE

If pain is a language, I have the accent on my tongue. I do not yet dream in pain, but an immersion has stripped my skeleton's previous fluency. Now I am a child in this land without good parking spaces.

(10:30) Today my husband and I talked about my calcified hip and aching hands, the awkwardness of a threesome with pain. We parked outside my therapist's office, claimed the flowered couch, and spoke about those ball-and-socket hips: so essential for knocking socks. The words came small, with squinting, like picking lice. A hundred geese cursed and laughed from the glinting marsh beyond the open window.

The therapist, who emails me pictures of her baby goats, asked me to describe the pain as a number. They never ask the pain's name, which could be Fucker or Bunny. Then: do you think you *are* the pain? I crunched my forehead to agonize in Venn diagrams: Am I coterminous with my disease? Overlapping?

It appeared that sex runways would have to be reconfigured, sex flight patterns remapped. The therapist smiled with optimism about the daunting industrial project of transferring a teenager's habit onto this irritable bag of Tinkertoys.

* * *

My body thinks you have rheumatoid arthritis.

Before the sex talk, at about 9:08 this morning, I saw my friend Jenny's picture on Facebook: dyed jet hair, three-quarter profile, sharp lips in a punk-rock smile as she held the drumsticks aloft.

Later (11:45) I parked alongside the yellow-orange, brick library and remembered the gold-tinged image of her. I winced: *Be careful not to hurt your wrists and shoulders with all that banging.* I saw in my mind a skeleton drummer, X-rayed with thick knots of danger.

No, wait—that's me. Not her. She's fine.

What grammar of disease operates beneath the surface of my skin and mind? As I called up the image, I reanimated Jenny with my own chemicals, crafted a tiny, diseased, punk-rock hazard. My body makes little bodies like itself.

I found Susan Sontag's *On Illness as Metaphor* in the library stacks; it was about cancer, T B, and I felt shamed to be complaining, grateful to have the language of lifespan.

I am neither well nor doomed. Sometimes I watch your soft bodies not in pain and can't remember. I push forward, each day of appointments a wager.

* * *

(12:30) The afternoon brought a kitchen-table meeting about assignments and syllabi along with an ache like rung metal. In two hours the January clouds had seeped into my joints in a diagonal drift from the west. I tasted a pressure system change: the flavors sharp or dull, the directions inward or out, pulsing like a northern lights I had mindlessly devoured.

Synovial fluid in my joints is inflamed in an autoimmune festival, my own personal Burning Woman, a conflagration semicontrolled with drugs but without cure.

One colleague, a rock-climber with enviable forearms and shoulders, sat across from me and talked Native American literature. I was distracted by the roaring of his body's utter silence, astounded as he angled fingers or turned a palm: he seemed to feel no pain, nor did he bargain with his skeleton. I wanted to interrupt the syllabi talk to ask whether he hurt anywhere, but I did not.

I am new at this; such ideas still run like a secret world underneath this one. I am at a child's level of pain-chatter. Later, perhaps, I will learn to constitute and imagine a range of bodies inside me as a child learns to imagine minds unlike her own. Maybe I will not always have to ask: can I show you mine, can I see yours?

* * *

(3:00) A final, hot-chocolate cafe meeting, free Wi-Fi and essay-talk, the writing itself a bliss of disembodied mind-union, but then I had pushed it too far.

(4:45) I pulled on E into a gas station and shut off the car with a pre-monition like a migraine aura: it's cresting. It wants more room. Freeze.

I closed my eyes to see it, big and stupid. The attention this morning made it bolder. My pain stretched out and preened like a stuffed lion with a Farrah Fawcett mane, proud and full of itself: *Ruffle my head.* How could I hate something so mute? Goddamn, floppy, aimless pain, unsightly as my pilled and grayed stuffed animals from childhood, those transitional objects so close to us they seem to have our faces, our first containers for love and for loss.

VI

MEASURING THE SKY

VITAL SIGN 5

"Meaningful functions" of chronic
pain for the body   0

Major systemic negative physiological
impacts of chronic pain   6

Percentage of world population in chronic pain   10–37

Percentage of U.S. population said to
be living with some form of chronic pain   47

Percentage estimated of pain population
in U.S. that is undertreated or untreated   30

Number of pain words making up a list in the
McGill Pain Scale, devised in 1975 to describe pain   78

Number of possibilities for describing pain
using the top section of the McGill Pain scale,
with options that allow a user to note pain
intensity and quality with 20 categories and
78 subcategories   233,280,000,000

Times I have been asked to use the McGill
Pain Scale to describe my own pain   0

Year when "Pain as the 5th Vital Sign" was
supported by the American Pain Society and then
adopted by the Veterans Health Administration   1996

Options for expressing pain using the
1–10 pain scale   10

Degree to which the 1–10 pain scale was
found to make a difference in terms of
treatment of chronic pain   0

Deaths in 2008 due to opioid overdoses   14,800

Percentage of opioid addicts who had their
painkillers prescribed by their doctor   18

Percentage of chronic pain patients who
get addicted to their pain pills   3–40

Number of patients in a systematic overview
of studies confirming that addiction is not a
major risk for chronic pain patients   88,235

Options I use in addition to pills for the
treatment of chronic pain   24

Percentage of chronic pain cases, in my humble
opinion, in which opioids should be discussed
as one option for short- or long-term treatment
under the supervision of a doctor   100

Profits made by Purdue Pharma in 2010
from the sale of OxyContin $3.1 billion

Odds of African Americans receiving no pain
medication compared to whites for a similar injury   63 percent greater

Cost to the U.S. each year of chronic pain in
terms of lost productivity and medical bills $635 billion

Number of Tramadol I took per day in
the summer of 2010 after my diagnosis   10

Number of hours it took me to begin weaning
myself off Tramadol after learning about its
decreasing efficacy   8

Number of times I have been addicted
to a medication   0

Times I have been shamed for following
doctors' orders with regard to taking an
opioid as prescribed by another doctor   3

Number of fucks I give about what doctors
think of me now and confidence I have in
most doctors' understanding of addiction
versus temporary chemical dependence   0

Times I have misspelled opioid   1,347

Specialists I have visited for a condition whose
primary symptom is chronic pain who did
not ask me a single question about how
I coped with chronic pain   7

Number of times I have developed a temporary
chemical dependence or tolerance to a medication
(including antidepressants) that disappeared after
a few weeks with minimal discomfort   4

Number of pain specialists in the
entire U.S. in 2011   4,000

ALTERNATIVE PAIN SCALE

When we go to see doctors and specialists, we are often asked to rate our pain on a 1 to 10 scale. I always get confused by this instrument, partly because I don't know what each level means. Is 1 "no pain," and would 10 be "the worst pain imaginable," such as being burned alive or torn limb from limb? Using that standard, it would seem arrogant for me to claim even an 8 if I was still able to function. So I use 1 to 7, with 7 being "bad," though I don't tell my doctor this. That puts my normal pain at 3, but I'm not sure how it helps my doctor if I repeat the number 3 over and over. So I have come up with a helpful replacement scale.

1. I have bold plans to revamp diet or try new stretches out of desperation borne by last night's pain, and I am overjoyed and energized that I am right now not in pain.
2. I'm busy-busy-busy, because if I move fast, the pain won't catch me! And I'm in motion now, but once I stop, I'll be drawn to the couch with magnetic force.
3. God, why am I so bitchy? Oh, wait—I'm in a sort of grinding, background-noise, world-clenching box of pain just beneath the edge of my conscious.
4. Couch. All I want is my couch and Netflix.
5. Wait, I'm kind of unsafe to drive just because I'm in pain. Like I can't think clearly. Wait: does that mean I'm high on pain itself?

Did I invent a free and unpleasant way to get high? Everything is suddenly funny. Pain Vegas!

6. Get the heat things and the cold things and the Tiger Balm and the various ointments and salves and put them all on me immediately.

7. Don't fucking touch me.

8. Do you still love me? Someone tell me they love me because I worry you hate me when I'm in pain. Am I irritating? Is it hard to love a near-invalid?

9. We need to check on our long-term disability policy. Do we have long-term disability? What if I can't work anymore? I can't go to work tomorrow but I have to. We need to make a Plan B right now. What about eel farming? Can we put eels in the pond behind your parents' house? Could we live on that? We should start buying cans of soup on sale and put them in the basement.

10. Everything is so beautiful and precious because I might die soon. I love that lampshade so very much.

11. I hate everyone, and everything is bothering me and making my skin feel gross, and I hate this couch where I've been lying for hours, and I just want a shower but the thought of the effort of a shower makes me want to cry.

12. I was born to play video games on my phone. I am good at this.

13. I can't read. The sentences are too hard. Remember when books?

14. I can't watch TV. I'll just scroll through Facebook in a fester of something unpleasant, but even the blue hurts my eyes. Look at all the healthy suckers doing things, completely oblivious to their looming deaths and physical disintegrations.

15. I can't even play games on my phone. My last stupid pleasure has been taken from me, and I wish to lodge a protest with the universe.

16. Where are the drugs? Oh—I stopped taking them because they wrecked my stomach. Where is that old bottle with the prescription from two years ago?

17. I don't even care about the drugs because I'm learning something from the pain. It's making me deep and spiritual, and I see shapes and colors. If I just roll with it, I can surf the pain. I can.

18. No, I'm not learning anything. I need the drugs, and the pain needs to be killed.

19. Mommy? Oh dammit I'm the mommy. Oh, just breathe like you're in labor. It will pass. (Except there's nothing good at the end, except maybe you will give birth to a horrible, gooey thing like in the movie Alien that will come and bite your face off.) Will someone please feel sorry for me immediately?

20. Am I going to puke? Would I feel better if I puked?

21. Words are hard. My name is . . . something? Whatever. "Name."

IN THE GRIP OF THE SKY

The sky has its way with me. As clouds lower their shoulders against the horizon, a warm front's humid body slides along my skin, lifting the hem of my dress to curl around my waist and stretch along my spine.

Closer still, the atmosphere enters me soundlessly. Barometric pressure squeezes my joints, each a tiny fishbowl of synovial fluid that cushions the space where two bones pivot and swing.

My immune system loves and defends me too diligently. I am one of the joint-diseased, we who have lupus and rheumatoid and psoriatic. If we could map our pain, the constellation of joints would glow on the map, lit to follow storm fronts and hurricanes. A joint-sick friend and I trade texts: *Rain coming—Got bad at 2 p.m., now flat on the couch. You?*

In this sky-grip I am one of many, and we are on fire.

I lie back, linked in pain with other bodies, in a kind of planetary transcendence. I watch the sky with closed eyes as an internal aurora borealis throbs, exquisite and strange. The rhythm and shifting whorls scrawl inside my flesh and bone in a patterned grammar I can almost pretend to decode. I have decided to listen to the air.

The inflamed atmosphere outside mirrors each tiny joint bubble inside me; the fates of both worlds have been permanently altered.

The heated sky skews and pitches, longing only for balance, hung with carbon-rich effluvia from the coal that launched Britain's navies and the factories of London. Outer and inner protective layers become inflamed. My overeager immune system works too well, devouring its host, while the planet's protective atmosphere holds the dangerous heat that men have made.

The atmospheric and the arthritic trace tendrils of smoke from the industrial explosion. My disease is said to be a signal miscopied, genes or molecules scrambled by chemical by-products that trace our desire to be faster and stronger than nature. My flesh and bones retract against the heat of the world's fever as the storms whip the planet's surface.

I and this pain-shadow lie on the couch. We turn in tandem under a blanket, as mare's tail clouds loop above me against the icy blue. If every body seated around the table at our climate negotiations had to push against a pain-shadow to stand or reach for a glass of water, to raise a hand to cast a vote, might each voice be raised in strong support for change? If every human felt the sky inside, we might wince against each turn of a key in an ignition. The islands being swallowed by water might seem not so far away.

In some minutes I feel beaten by the sky. Bobbing down, my spirit fights for air. I have learned to push up into this pain storm out of curiosity and a need to understand. Each throb reminds me of my permeability. The gases surrounding our planet follow every move I make, pushing at my nerves. I sometimes shake my fist at the sky, but I do not hate the clouds; I do not hate them even when they seem to deliver terrible blows. Their impact is a desperate appeal, intending to reach us, even as far as under the skin, to drag us to safety.

BETWEEN ONE AND TEN THOUSAND

Philosopher Elaine Scarry writes that pain resists speech and expression; a person in pain is certain of the pain, but anyone hearing about the pain has only doubt or questions: "Unseeable classes of objects such as subterranean plates, Seyfert galaxies, and the pains occurring in other people's bodies flicker before the mind, then disappear."

One adjective will not do for pain. Sometimes when I watch pain in my body, it feels very disaggregated, like one of those lumpy casseroles from my midwestern childhood with chunks of meat and green beans, held in place with a coating of viscous cream of mushroom soup, topped with the fried onions that are sold in a paper can.

This sense of pain as an aggregate comforts me; I see it as part of my job of being in pain to let the pain itself come into focus, to pay attention to it, so its strands and colors become distinct and, therefore, less overwhelming. I am kind of a park ranger of pain. I throw metaphors at it. I gesture-draw rapid sketches, because pain hungers for representation of itself.

"Physical pain does not simply resist language but actively destroys it," Scarry writes, "bringing about an immediate reversion to a state anterior to language, to the sounds and cries a human being makes before language is learned." One of Scarry's subjects is the horrific and specific pain of torture, the aim of which is to dehumanize, to render nonverbal and insensate. My pain is thankfully not this severe, so I am sometimes in the gray zone between language and non-language. Yet, although pain sometimes makes me nonverbal, it does not reduce me to a state before image. I see solid objects and colors when I am in pain, as if pain longs for form. As I was transcribing quotes from Scarry's book, my husband asked me a question, and it took work to formulate an answer. I saw a large clear block, something like a huge, old television, and I had to climb laboriously up onto it in my mind in order to gain access to language. It was tiring, but I opened my mouth and made sentences. Even in those few seconds where I was technically, momentarily nonverbal, I had image and color, the building blocks in children's minds that are even older than speech and that represent the world.

Pain is sometimes a muting firewall that separates me from the files and scripts of my personality. I have the directory remaining but none of the contents. Sometimes pain blunts my memory of myself. On those days I reach into the toolbox of my head blindly, grasping and hoping I can make "Sonya" do what is expected of "Sonya" in social situations. Even in those moments, I look for the texture of the muting. I pay attention to the way my muted mind grasps toward the memory of small talk.

In old Taoist and Zen texts, the stuff of reality was referred to as the "ten thousand things." If you imagine the world—all of its crazy bits and pieces and gears and butterfly wings and catalytic converters, each interacting in subtle ways with everything else—you get the sense of a vast net. Touch one point, and the whole thing ripples. This is the Buddhist concept of the interconnected nature of reality. The word *Tathata* in Sanskrit is often translated as "suchness," the textured "this-ness" of the world. This textured net also connects to the idea of karma, because it follows that one action would affect the whole net.

Before I needed the net and the metaphors, pain from a skinned knee or a pulled muscle radiated along nerve signals to my brain, from periphery to center. I could ice the skin, rub the muscle, and wince at the world's incursion on my body. Even depression had a location; I could feel it swirling in my brain. Rheumatoid arthritis is systemic, so it hurts all over. The pain is everywhere, and, therefore, in a strange way it is in danger of being a nothing, background noise, expanding like space to envelop and subsume me.

My pain began in my joints, those tiny, saltwater fishbowls of synovial fluid meant to buffer our movement, the fantastic invention of the earthbound mammals. I believe our joints are the pockets of memories from our underwater life. I remember distinctly the moment when I gripped the steering wheel in my car and had to admit that something was wrong with mine; it should not have been so hard to move those digits, the five-splayed mark of humankind. Within me a barely understood autoimmune process had caused my body to attack itself, beginning with those synovial pockets. The pain might spread to connective tissue, to permanently aggravated nerves, and to various weakened organs. Pain compounds health problems because it tempts the sufferer to move as little as possible, as if to allow the beast to sleep.

Chronic pain comes in two flavors. Hyperalgesia is an exaggerated response to something that hurts, so a pinprick feels like a hammer blow. Allodynia is a pain feeling caused by something that wouldn't normally hurt, like the touch of a bed sheet. Different nerve cells function to relay these pain versus non-pain signals, but it's believed that both types are sensitized to repeated pain signals, essentially getting better at their jobs in response to increased information. Think about this: our neural networks branch out beautifully in response to stimuli, and our brains' real estate expands to encompass what we are good at. This is a problem for chronic pain patients, whose nervous systems become shaped into balls of fire that attempt, over and over, to interpret an internal sensation as an external threat.

Because my pain has no external expression other than a few gently twisting knuckles, it depends upon me for expression and metaphor. In fact, if I don't feed it metaphor on a daily basis, my pain devours me. It may gobble me up anyway through disease process, inflammation, and mental decline associated with the stress of chronic pain. But I have this belief, based upon years of experience, that the more metaphor I can feed my pain, the better chance I have of maintaining the thread of lucid thought as I navigate within it and it navigates within me.

Scarry again: "The only state that is as anomalous as pain is the imagination. While pain is a state remarkable for being wholly without objects, the imagination is remarkable for being the only state that is wholly its objects." Scarry means that pain is a completely internal and invisible experience; imagination is the finding of internal representations so that the imagined can be expressed to one's self or others.

My pain digs up the most colorful, garish analogies. Its 1970s taste is all polyester, Day-Glo, and black-lit space opera. It wants purple eye shadow or else it wants to become every muscled beast. In fact, it seems to want everything I can't be anymore: racing, screaming, go-go dancing, raving. It is terrained, one metaphor after another, metaphors inside metaphors, bubbles of worlds that develop and pop. But each is free, none requires a co-pay, and if they are addictive then so be it. Let my pain shape itself into worlds. It fancies itself quite wild, many-eyed, but somehow bluish and gentle, living where the wild things are yet waiting for comfort and visits from children in jammies. My pain digs up the dregs of me, the way-back scraps from childhood stories and the rawest threads of self, in order to make signals and tell me what it is. It wants nothing more than to speak, and I honestly believe it does not want to do me harm.

But why give this pain voice or consciousness, and why imagine it as a character? Pain once was mere impulse within me, flashes of functional telegraph signals. But when it became chronic, it began to live a continued existence. Who can say that it has not found a kind of consciousness within me purely because its presence has become sustained through inflammation and the way that chronic pain feeds on itself, ringing its own bells? Pain finds itself alive in me, born without asking to have been conceived. In my personal mythology I believe pain is searching for a way to harm me as little as possible, asking for language and image to minimize its impact, hoping that interpretation will lead to ease and a kind of coexistence.

Now as I lie on the couch with the laptop on my lap, pain throbs within my second row of knuckles like a clacking of castanets, while the cradle of my hips hums a bass throb. My knees whine a sharp minor note, which echoes back to my hips, and my shoulders want somehow to push outward from this carapace in a clear oboe call, paralleled by the trill of my cervical spine, just a touched note. And in response to these sharp notes there's the soft burr of a headache, the hurt I don't really even sense immediately, the background white noise of muscle groups tensing in response to the nerve signals from the joints. Some of the hip pain is probably lower back muscles, and if I were to get very careful, push through the loud chords of knee and hip, I would be able to sense the softer aches in the hamstrings and the calves. I check in with the ankles and for a moment find them silent, my toes happily mute.

I absorb solace in podcasts on Buddhist philosophy and meditation that I listen to on the drive to work. I learn about the net of interdependence and the way in which solidifying concepts leads to pain.

This idea matters to me only because it has changed my world. As I watch the shifting pain inside me, I know that pain will continue to shift and flow rather than solidify. If it waxes, it will wane, and that is hope. If it moves, it is not an anvil crushing me. It is not a demon with a consistent texture. Its shiftiness requires the kinds of metaphors that stress its aggregate nature. Its aggregate nature keeps me sane, because it is not a battle of me versus pain as an abstract presence but instead me very much alive watching what pain does, what it really is from moment to moment. Pain drapes uneasily over my skeleton, or maybe even easily some days, as if it loves me. It is me, after all, just not in the form I would like my components to take.

Scarry writes that pain can be a "wholly passive and helpless occur-rence," until a person in pain actively engages the imagination in rela-tion to the pain. At this point pain becomes "an intentional state" that can be "self-modifying and, when most successful, self-eliminating."

As a writer, I have been slowly trained to love the details of the world as a key to technical and narrative excellence, so it is not surprising that such a view would also become a container for spiritual focus and a way to manage physical discomfort. In his writing George Orwell drew the observed details into sharp focus, steering away from the abstractions he saw as connected to the dulling effects of political doublespeak. A review of a volume of Orwell's diaries noted his devotion to the "thinginess" of life.

The ancient Greek word for "ten thousand" is mu, represented by M, and the word root in Greek is connected to the word for "myriad" in English.

On some mornings, the very word "thinginess" makes me misty-eyed with reverence. I am here, in the thinginess itself, and I used to be far-away in the ocean of abstraction, of concepts and would and when and then. Pain is purely in the present, like a Buddhist koan. Memories of pain are dulled or blotted out, signified in red ink in the brain rather than re-created. When we are in pain, we are in the now, so the net I live inside is the essence of life as it is happening.

This does not make me "grateful" for the pain—though honestly I do not know anymore what anyone means by "gratitude" because of the word's ubiquity and commercialization. Pain requires me to be present in order to track it, so that is my job description. Pain has an edge and a clear danger. Mentally it triggers fear and the gray mist of depression, so pain must be uncovered to the pale roots before sadness lodges in and grows, before I lose the insight that pain might be triggering my doom, my distrust of people, and the day itself. Physically it can lead one to stay in bed, which weakens the body and its ability to connect with others and withstand pain. I don't know whether I'm grateful for pain; I don't think that's relevant.

Pain is not a Jesus that wants anything from me. It doesn't scold or wag its finger, doesn't judge, and doesn't give a shit how its human handles itself. It just is, like the Grand Canyon, not as a concept or a postcard but the square inches that together find themselves forming a crater without specific consciousness of their outline. Sometimes my metaphors collide; in this one, pain doesn't understand itself.

Sosan, the Third Japanese Zen Patriarch, 606 CE, wrote in *The Book of True Faith* that meditation is a state in which the subject and the object are not separated; "Each contains itself and the ten thousand things."

Pain is a windshield with nerves, and I have to scrape it raw to see beyond myself. Trees and buildings smudge behind the ice sheet of pain. I miss so much of what is said, and the sky seems lowered like an eyelid.

Or pain is the weather itself, a crashing, raining thing, soaking me so completely that I can't even figure out its source. Again it is something like having a sieve on my head; pain fragments my vision and makes the sound tinny. The images proliferate and shift.

According to Scarry, we are all living between the bookends of pain and imagination, which are the "framing events" of life. Between them, "all other perceptual, somatic, and emotional events occur; thus, between the two extremes can be mapped the whole terrain of the human psyche."

The experimental musician John Cage, who was also heavily influenced by Zen, composed an experimental piece called *The Ten Thousand Things*. In a letter to a friend, he described this piece as "a large work which will always be in progress and will never be finished; at the same time any part of it will be able to be performed once I have begun. It will include tape and any other time actions, not excluding violins and whatever else I put my attention to . . ." He envisioned the song as a composite of multiple pieces, with instructions for sampling them in specific intervals that would recompose with each new hearing. This morning, with pain ebbing in a crest across my shoulder bones, fluted like a piecrust or the frill of a ceratopsian dinosaur, tears prick in my ducts at the thought of John Cage creating and naming a work that will never be done. Pain is not a project or a product. I try to simplify and manage it, underestimating it, taking off slices and opening it up. I try to wrap it up, and it soaks through the wrapping.

Pain is a screaming infant I must attend to before anything else. To assess the cause of discomfort, I must collect the details of a harsh cry and reddened face or thrashing limbs, even as I navigate around the tension of the noise and the confusion, exhaustion, and frustration. Parenting this pain is the act of steering myself back from the future, the abstract fears over whether I will be able to handle it, to raise it, or to let it go. Pain, like parenting, is real only in the moments that make up its whole.

The ten thousand things can be a snare to catch me if I fixate on it as separate from myself or see the world in a dualistic way and push against it. My mind wants easy divisions: me versus it, good versus bad. I push against the binary because that is my job. This pain is not bad; it just is. I return to the neutral place at the middle of the web between bouts of intense struggle with the sticky threads of the ten thousand things.

I made a sketch a few years ago that hung above my desk at work, one of those concept bubble charts where ideas appear in circles, and you draw lines to connect ideas that seem to resonate with each other. The "ten thousand things" appeared in a bubble and also seemed to describe the web itself.

Each neuron in the brain is supposed to be connected to ten thousand others.

There's no telling exactly what sparked this disease. Some say that autoimmune diseases increase based on childhood stresses, and those childhood stresses ripple backward through their own causes in my family tree. If exposure to chemical contamination has sparked the pain, which chemical and which open pore of contact? Or maybe it is partly the messages of genetics. I am a wild and inscrutable process, an expression of the fiery universe itself with supernovas. My cells have received garbled instructions, unhelpful directives, and who among us has not been charged by an employer with an irrational task? My parts are doing the best they can.

Scarry writes that when a person makes images out of her pain, she creates "not the shape of the skeleton, the shape of the body weight, nor even the shape of pain-perceived, but the shape of perceived-pain-wished-gone." Only in this regard do I disagree with her. While I long for my pain to be gone, the pain-shapes in my mind are not hateful. At least so far I continue to be curious about the pain, and I feel almost as though I must watch it carefully to continue to know it, to collect data, to keep pace with it, to track it and see what it turns into next. I am curious about this overlapping pain body, which is still a part of my internal universe. The metaphors I choose for pain are never violent, which may be part of the imagination working to transform inchoate suffering into the humble and mundane objects of the world.

These days "me" is quite permeable. Without help in the form of doctors, supplements, medications, family members, and supportive friends, I might disintegrate rapidly, so "me" is loose and expansive. My body requires a net of ten thousand things and is no longer contained within its own skin. I used to see this as weakness, but I can also see it as permeability. When I get ready to go to sleep, I take four or five pills. I turn on an air filter for my allergies and bite down on a clear, hard, plastic mouth guard to soothe my jaw joint pain. I put an earplug in each ear to shore up my shallow pool of sleep, smooth moisturizer on my hands, lip balm on my lips, and lavender essential oil on my wrists and temples. I lean my head back on a squishy pillow that supports my cervical spine and place another pillow between my knees. I covet sleep because it works better than any drug to help the body rebound from pain.

Coming into contact with pain is not leaving myself but instead affirming that I am part of it and everything else. The great Master Dogen said, "To study the Buddha Way is to study the self, to study the self is to forget the self, and to forget the self is to be enlightened by the ten thousand things."

In another story from the Tang dynasty, a government official and a Zen master named Nansen strolled together in a garden. The official quoted the Zen monk Sosan, who said, "The ten-thousand things and I are of one substance." Nansen pointed at a garden where they were strolling and replied, "People look at these flowers as if they were in a dream." In other words (I think) we mull over the beauty of the flowers, but what is more extraordinary is that we are part of them, not actually separate from them at all, and this is the bad dream of separation in which we are trapped.

What did it feel like not to be in pain? I can't say I remember. But I don't always actively hate this existence. It's me. I like me. This is part of it. Some people run marathons, searching for the extensive mental and physical challenge that I get by lying on the couch. They get to wear numbers on their chests, and they affix stickers on the back of their car with numbers describing the length of a marathon. I do the same physical, creative, adaptive, nonverbal, focused, deep-breathing, minute-to-minute practice every single day. My marathon comes with me wherever I go.

Coming into communion with pain can be scary, because it requires me to open my skull. Sometimes I'd rather avoid it with candy and Facebook, and I'd rather stay in control. The first few minutes of letting go are free fall. I lie down and close my eyes. I must orient myself in deep space. When I tumble into it, there's a sense of falling, and then my body becomes three-dimensional and intelligible, and I can sense dull clusters of things besides the pain.

Some nights the pain is like the thumb of God right on me. There is no managing pain when it gets to this point of being a starry sky, and the only choice I have is supplication. The passion is the exact location where one's boundaries dissolve, like the loneliness and grandeur of camping on an ice field. I am a Buddhist, and yet I feel God in that faceless contact, as if I am standing below the expanse of the Milky Way, beneath the lit array, in awe of something vast, universal, other than human.

INSIDE THE NAUTILUS

The body itself is a screen
to shield and partially reveal
the light that's blazing
inside your presence.

    —Rumi, "Story Water"

Measure a dream. Map the far-flung geography of a night's restless searching. Compare the longing or love of today with the homesickness you felt a year ago. The answers are poems that pool and slip between my fingers.

Pain is the body's nightmare. The body pulls back the edges of her mouth, and the brain fogs. The hands wave in vague circles, point to problem areas, and the eyes search the floor, the ceiling. When words fail, we turn to numbers. A doctor hands me a piece of paper with charts and diagrams. The paper asks me to repeat all the information I think I know: name, date of birth, address, diagnosis. Like syllables repeated so often, they unspool into nonsense, the data to denote self becomes unhinged from its referent. The blanks on these forms fog my sense of self: who is this throbbing creature? I am disembodied and flat like the naked, hairless outline of the cartoon man on the form, depicted standing or lying from the front and then flipped to his back like a pancake. I am instructed to circle the places on his body that correspond to my hurt. The man has blank circles for pupils, and he seems compliant and resigned to his fate, yet he is muscled and perfectly symmetrical.

I must do well on this form because it is my only chance to let the pain speak. I press my lips together, looking back and forth between the form and an internal space, listening for pain's tracks. Was it worse a week ago? How would I rate my overall health compared to yesterday, last week, last month?

How would *you* rate your overall health compared to a month ago at this time? Would it be a three on a scale of one to ten, or slightly more? Does your existence rank a seven?

No matter what I choose, the body shifts, rankles, resigns itself to a grade that does not fit its effort, its hope, its depression, its fever dream, or its beauty.

Yet doctors must ask, because qualitative data must tether to a baseline so that a treatment plan can be created and so that progress or decline may be noted. Forms for charting pain include the Visual Analogue Scale, the Neuropathic Pain Scale, the Numerical Rating Scale, the Brief Pain Inventory, the Faces Pain Scale, or the Verbal Descriptor Scale. A study by Dr. Y. Yazici Sayin comparing these methods revealed that most patients felt "their pain was not measured with any of the pain scales."

I have rated my pain on the one to ten pain scale (NRS) more times than I can count. I have circled and compared and then handed over the clipboard with hopelessness, knowing I'm underrating and not adequately expressing the pain. I know that women tend to underreport pain, as do rheumatoid patients. But I have not been in another body; I only know this pain could be worse. On a one to five scale, I don't allow myself to go above a three unless it's a true emergency. I save nine for the feelings of childbirth and being drawn and quartered, so eight must be the limit before losing consciousness.

My doctors tally up the results, enter the number in my file, and the form disappears, another page in my body of work.

After five years of filling out these forms, and a few hours of researching them, I came across the McGill Pain Questionnaire. I scanned the instructions and began to consider the first table, which asked "What Does Your Pain Feel Like?

Had I ever been personally addressed by a form? Here, at least, I was a "you," a being as well as a named body. And "feel"—one's heart might catch in one's throat at that very word, capacious and wide, capturing that squishy acknowledgment that this was a demanding act of translation.

The table before me offered a transfixing list of words in categories that only a person in pain would know. The category "brightness" asked me to choose among the ranked options of *itchy, tingling, smarting,* and *stinging.* I chose itchy, and it was accurate. Pain has a kind of brightness when it seems to float to the surface and almost want to rise above my skin. And it has dullness when it seems to sink deep toward my bones. We don't give pain this nuance and credit, tending to portray it as bricks of solid sensation, but it has its own palette. I began to move down the rows, considering and composing my poem.

Another category seemed to rank the pain as its pulse beat against one's body, like music, with options, including *flickering* and *pounding.* Other questions tracked pain's spatial location and its heat. The category "punishment" listed these adjectives as choices: *punishing, grueling, cruel, vicious,* and *killing.* As frightening as these words might seem, I read this list and felt the muscles around my sternum loosen in relief. The syllables in their order named a voiceless void, transforming suffering into a hallway within the building of human culture. I suspected that even filling out this form created a measurable clinical benefit in my physical/mental body, as if hope of a common language itself might ease this body's struggle against itself.

I followed the directions, choosing adjectives only in categories I felt in that moment and skipping categories that were not true in that slice of time. I received this string of adjectives: *Throbbing, flashing, drilling, sharp, crushing, pulling, hot, itchy, sore, tiring, troublesome, penetrating, squeezing,* and *nagging*. Each adjective had a point value, so I added them up and received a number: thirty-four.

I began to love this poet-healer McGill. I savored the form with a quiet outpouring of affection one reserves for sensitive thinkers and researchers whose work plumbs the core of human experience. Yet as with any poem, there was so much white space in the margins. I ached for this unknown doctor who I imagined must have received a grievous injury or borne an insidious disease, because there was no other way he could know these secret things.

I want to make a needlepoint for McGill, maybe, or raisin bread.

I moved to the section "How does your pain change over time?" and answered questions about how it is right now (discomforting), how it is at its worst and least (excruciating and mild). I ranked my worst rheumatoid pain at a five, and the worst toothache or stomachache at a four. I followed the instructions and added up a total of sixteen for this section. The brilliance of this form was that it asked for a long-term perspective; all the other forms seem to care only about how I was doing right at that moment or over the last week, which is not an accurate snapshot of the pain experience.

After adding the three sections, I determined a combined McGill of fifty out of seventy-eight. It was mine, this pain. My pain was strong. I have sometimes seen my pain as a foreign force that has bested me, laid me low, and never as though I were a container, holding this fifty, balancing this throbbing crystal vase of pain on my head and ably continuing.

I turned to Wikipedia to learn that there was no McGill to fall in love with—or rather, that the scale was called McGill because it was created at McGill University in Canada. It was created by Ronald Melzack and W. S. Torgerson, first published in 1975, building on Melzack's research and time spent listening to people in pain.

While in school for his doctorate, Melzack began to work with amputee patients who had phantom limb syndrome, a particular pain that agonized and persisted despite having little external expression in the tissue. He began collecting "pain words" from his patients, and later he put them into groups that seemed to belong together.

He sought out more people in pain and listened. His form came from the mouths of people in pain as they searched for words to describe their experience. The form—in addition to being accurate and poetic—is scientifically reliable and reproducible. It's been translated into fifty languages and found to be statistically valid and meaningful across cultures. Around the world, people tended to use the same words to describe their pain. This is my dream of a common language.

I googled "I love Ron Melzack" as though I were scrawling the sentence on a folder in high school. It turned out that no one on the Internet has written the phrase. I was sad again that Melzack's form had never found its way to me via a doctor. I cast backward and outward, imagining a world and a country in particular where doctors would have time or inclination to consider this form's data worthwhile.

I wanted to see Dr. Melzack's face, so I searched for pictures. I studied his image, an older, balding man with a long face and a nice, thoughtful smile. His shoulders sloped, as if he were tall and used to stooping. I found a video from McGill University. Upon learning that he was still alive, I briefly considered a road trip, but decide it would be creepy to drive to Canada to say thank you to a scholar of pain.

In the video he sat in his office describing his research. The orderly spiral of a bisected nautilus shell hung in a frame on the wall behind him, that proportioned geometry from nature expressing the golden mean and the promise of logical construction to a creature's development. The nautilus reminded me of Melzack's form, its compartments providing safety and structure. Melzack described his early research with dogs in pain, which led him to the idea that a person's prior experience would shape how they interpreted pain. His theory—that pain was a complex constellation involving the brain, the nerves, and the emotions—flew in the face of centuries of simple theories of pain, beginning with René Descartes's idea that pain was a message that traveled up a nerve to the brain.

The interviewer on the video asked, "Why pain?"

Melzack smiled shyly and described his credo for research: "Pick a tough problem. Don't pick an easy one. The joy of research is the challenge of the problem."

Inspired by his continuing work with phantom limb pain, in the early 1990s he developed the neuromatrix theory, which describes a map of one's body contained in one's brain. He let another shy smile escape and said, "I have the neuromatrix theory. What I don't have is a model of the brain that would fit it. So what I'm developing is a new way of looking at the brain."

In his modest office, in front of a painted, white cinderblock wall with the careful slow record of a nautilus's work behind him, he was asked how it felt to be on the trail of something so huge and to have accomplished so much. "It's very gratifying," he said. "It's wonderful, and it makes me want to continue, because the job isn't all done."

During a day in which I lay on the couch, and pain occluded my thinking, I lingered in the world of YouTube and fell into a two-hour video about the latest science of pain, all research building on Melzack's foundational work. I learned about the complex bundles of nerves that carry different kinds of signals and how each is triggered by a different type of pain. I learned about nerve sheaths and allodynia, hyperalgesia, neuropathy, and tissue damage. The science provided a massive comfort for one female neuromatrix and physical body trying to find meaning and order, enfolding me like the segments of a shell.

The researcher on the video, Dr. Allan Basbaum, turned from his PowerPoint slides and said to his students in the lecture hall, "As far as I'm concerned, if there's no emotional response, there's no pain." In other words, pain is upsetting. He added, "Pain is not a stimulus. Pain is an emotional experience."

Basbaum clicked to a slide of two horribly deformed hands of a rheumatoid arthritis patient. He explained something surprising but completely understandable to me, which was that while mauled hands are difficult for patients to adapt to, these patients consistently report the pain itself is far worse than any deformity. Not being able to do things with agility is a challenge, but movement in which each second is painful is a greater obstacle.

Over and over, doctors have regarded my body to look for the non-verbal, the nonemotional, checking my hands and feet to see minimal deformity. They have called me "lucky" because the body's outward signals, as mute as a nautilus shell's smooth surface, cannot speak about the sharp and segmented poetry within.

SOURCES

Biss, Eula. "The Pain Scale," *Harper's Magazine*, June 2005.

Broyard, Anatole. *Intoxicated by My Illness and Other Writings on Life and Death.* New York: Fawcett, 1993.

Felstiner, Mary. *Out of Joint: A Private and Public Story of Arthritis.* Lincoln: University of Nebraska Press, 2007.

Foreman Judy. *A Nation in Pain: Healing Our Biggest Health Problem.* New York: Oxford University Press, 2014.

Frank, Arthur W. *The Wounded Storyteller: Body, Illness, and Ethics,* 2nd edition, 79–81. Chicago: University of Chicago Press, 2013.

Hamblyn, Richard. *The Invention of Clouds.* New York: Farrar, Straus & Giroux, 2001.

Haraway, Donna. "A Manifesto for Cyborgs: Science, Technology, and Socialist Feminism." In *Feminism/Postmodernism,* edited by Linda J. Nicholson. New York: Routledge, 1990.

Lorde, Audre. *The Cancer Journals,* special edition. San Francisco: Aunt Lute Books, 2006.

Lorde, Audre, and Joan Wylie Hall. *Conversations with Audre Lorde.* Jackson: University Press of Mississippi, 2004.

Mairs, Nancy. *Waist-High in the World: A Life among the Non-Disabled.* Boston: Beacon Press, 1997.

Malham, David. "Memento Mori." *New York Times,* March 11, 2015.

Montaigne, Michel de. *The Complete Essays.* New York: Penguin, 2004.

Rapp, Emily. *Poster Child.* New York: Bloomsbury, 2008.

Scarry, Elaine. *The Body in Pain: The Making and Unmaking of the World.* New York: Oxford University Press, 1987.

Sontag, Susan. *On Illness as Metaphor and AIDS and Its Metaphors.* New York: Picador, 2001.

———. *Regarding the Pain of Others.* New York: Picador, 2004.

Weeks, Kathi. *The Problem with Work: Feminism, Marxism, Antiwork Politics and Postwork Imaginaries*, p. 54. Durham: Duke University Press, 2011.

THE STATUS OF PAIN

Charlotte Bohnett, "Social Media: A Valuable Health Resource for Patients." *WebPT*, July 2, 2012.

INTERSTATE AND INTERBEING

The notion of interbeing comes from Thich Nhat Hahn, *How to Love* (Berkeley: Parallax Press, 2014).

VITAL SIGN 5

0: "Chronic pain serves no meaningful purpose for the body," from Anthony J. Alvarado, "Cultural Diversity: Pain Beliefs and Treatment among Mexican Americans, African-Americans, Chinese-Americans, and Japanese-Americans." Nursing honors thesis, Eastern Michigan University, 2008. http://commons.emich.edu/cgi/viewcontent.cgi?article=1126&context =honors.

6: P. G. Fine, "Long-term Consequences of Chronic Pain: Mounting Evidence for Pain as Neurological Disease and Parallels with Other Chronic Disease States." *Pain Medicine.* 12, no. 7 (July 2011):996–1004. "Including sleep, cognitive processes and brain function, mood/mental health, cardiovascular health, sexual function, and overall quality of life. Furthermore, chronic pain has the capacity to become increasingly complex in its pathophysiology, and thus potentially more difficult to treat over time. The various health complications related to chronic pain can also incur significant economic consequences for patients."

10: Tracy P. Jackson, MD, Victoria Sutton Stabile, K.A. Kelly McQueen. "The Global Burden of Chronic Pain." *American Society of Anesthesiologists* 78, no. 6 (June 1, 2014): 24

37: Philip A. Pizzo, et al., *Relieving Pain in America: A Blueprint for Transforming Prevention, Care, Education, and Research*. Institute of Medicine (U.S.) Committee on Advancing Pain Research, Care, and Education. Washington DC: National Academies Press, 2011.

47: Alyssa Brown, "Chronic Pain Rates Shoot Up until Americans Reach Late 50s," *Gallup*. April 27, 2012. Lower-income people were significantly more likely to experience chronic pain.

30: Foreman, *A Nation in Pain*, 137

78: https://www.gem-beta.org/public/DownloadMeasure.aspx?mid=1348.

233,280,000,000: My own math. Could very well be wrong.

1996: Department of Veterans Affairs. "Take 5: Pain as the 5th Vital Sign," October 2000 revised edition. It was recommended in 1999 that pain be measured on a one to ten scale as the "fifth vital sign," a practice that began in Veterans Administration Hospitals and became widespread. http://www.va.gov/PAINMANAGEMENT/docs/Pain_As_the_5th_Vital_Sign_Toolkit.pdf.

10: It's true.

0: Richard A. Mularski, MD, MSHS; Foy White-Chu, MD; Devorah Overbay, MS, RN; Lois Miller, PhD, RN,4; Steven M Asch, MD, MPH,1,2; and Linda Ganzini, MD, MPH, "Measuring Pain as the 5th Vital Sign Does Not Improve Quality of Pain Management," Journal of General Internal Medicine 21, no. 6 (June 2006):607–12. "Patients ($n=79$) who reported substantial pain often did not receive recommended care: 22% had no attention to pain documented in the medical record, 27% had no further assessment documented, and 52% received no new therapy for pain at that visit."

14,800: United States Senate Committee on Finance, "Baucus, Grassley Seek Answers about Opioid Manufacturers' Ties to Medical Groups," May 8, 2012.

18: Miranda Hitti, "Prescription Painkiller Addiction: 7 Myths." WebMD. 57 percent said they'd received the pills from someone they knew, according to a 2007 survey. Doing the math, this means that patients themselves are not the addicts, in the majority of cases.

3–40: "Chronic Pain Treatment and Addiction." National Institute on Drug Abuse, 2014. This is not well studied, and addiction itself is difficult to study. One study found that 5 percent who take the prescriptions as directed become addicted: "Opioids and Chronic Pain." National Institutes of Health MedlinePlus, Spring 2011.

88,235: Jennifer Van Pelt, "Pain Care Advocacy in an Era of Opioid Abuse." *Social Work Today* 12, no. 5:16. In other words, scientists re-examined all the studies on addiction and pain and confirmed that addiction is not a major risk for the majority of pain patients; the total number of patients in these studies is 88,235.

24: I use these non-opioid treatments for chronic pain: Meditation three times a week but should be seven, turmeric, boswellia, lavender oil, exercise at hopefully ten thousand steps a day, nine hours of sleep, mouth guard, special neck pillow, earplugs, pillow between the knees, neti pot for nasal inflammation, air filter for allergies, gluten-free diet for treatment of inflammation, egg-free for treatment of inflammation, soy-free for treatment of inflammation, acupuncture, stretches, massage, rest, social life limitation, cane, supportive fingerless arthritis gloves, arnica lotion, and Tiger Balm.

3.1: Meredith Tracey, "Five Pharmaceutical Companies Sued in Response to Opioid Addiction Epidemic." PM360, July 15, 2014. Purdue Pharma and four other companies were the target of a lawsuit claiming that they over-marketed opioids to vulnerable populations; this is what we have instead of an organized medical response to pain.

63: Pizzo, *Relieving Pain in America*.

$635 billion: Pizzo, *Relieving Pain in America*.

4,000: Maia Szalavitz, "Chronic, Undertreated Pain Affects 116 Million Americans." *Time*. June 29, 2016.

BETWEEN ONE AND TEN THOUSAND

Barry Gewen, "Staying Power," a review of George Orwell's diaries. *New York Times Book Review*, September 2, 2012.

Hsin-hsin Ming, *Faith Mind Inscription.* www.sacred-texts.com/bud/zen
/fm/fm.htm.

James Pritchett, *The Music of John Cage.* New York: Cambridge University
Press, 1996.

Eihei Dogen, *The Way of Everyday Life: Zen master Dogen's Genjokoan.* Los
Angeles: Zen Center of Los Angeles, 1978.

INSIDE THE NAUTILUS

Allan I. Basbaum, MD. "The Science of Pain," University of California Television. March 15, 2012. Accessed October 26, 2015. https://www.youtube
.com/watch?v=-TN1r25wAoI.

Tatsuyuki Arimura, "Pain Questionnaire Development Focusing on Cross-
Cultural Equivalence to the Original Questionnaire: The Japanese Version
of the Short-Form McGill Pain Questionnaire" *Pain Medicine* 13, no. 4
(April 1, 2012): 541–51.

"Ronald Melzack: Pain Pioneer." McGill University, uploaded October 6, 2010.
Accessed October 26, 2015. https://www.youtube.com/watch?v=KRFan
GInvlc.

Yazile Yazici Sayin, et al. "Comparison of Pain Scale Preferences and Pain
Intensity According to Pain Scales among Turkish Patients: A Descriptive
Study." *Pain Management Nursing* 15, no. 1 (March 1, 2014): 156–64.

IN THE AMERICAN LIVES SERIES

Fault Line
by Laurie Alberts

Pieces from Life's Crazy Quilt
by Marvin V. Arnett

Songs from the Black Chair:
A Memoir of Mental Illness
by Charles Barber

This Is Not the Ivy League:
A Memoir
by Mary Clearman Blew

Body Geographic
by Barrie Jean Borich

Driving with Dvořák:
Essays on Memory and Identity
by Fleda Brown

Searching for Tamsen Donner
by Gabrielle Burton

Island of Bones: Essays
by Joy Castro

American Lives: A Reader
edited by Alicia Christensen
introduced by Tobias Wolff

Get Me Through Tomorrow:
A Sister's Memoir of Brain
Injury and Revival
by Mojie Crigler

Should I Still Wish: A Memoir
by John W. Evans

Out of Joint: A Private and
Public Story of Arthritis
by Mary Felstiner

Descanso for My Father:
Fragments of a Life
by Harrison Candelaria Fletcher

My Wife Wants You to Know
I'm Happily Married
by Joey Franklin

Weeds: A Farm
Daughter's Lament
by Evelyn I. Funda

Falling Room
by Eli Hastings

Opa Nobody
by Sonya Huber

Pain Woman Takes Your Keys, and
Other Essays from a Nervous System
by Sonya Huber

Hannah and the Mountain: Notes
toward a Wilderness Fatherhood
by Jonathan Johnson

Local Wonders: Seasons in
the Bohemian Alps
by Ted Kooser

Bigger than Life:
A Murder, a Memoir
by Dinah Lenney

What Becomes You
by Aaron Raz Link
and Hilda Raz

*Queen of the Fall: A Memoir
of Girls and Goddesses*
by Sonja Livingston

Such a Life
by Lee Martin

Turning Bones
by Lee Martin

In Rooms of Memory: Essays
by Hilary Masters

Between Panic and Desire
by Dinty W. Moore

Sleep in Me
by Jon Pineda

*The Solace of Stones: Finding
a Way through Wilderness*
by Julie Riddle

*Works Cited: An Alphabetical
Odyssey of Mayhem and
Misbehavior*
by Brandon R. Schrand

Thoughts from a Queen-Sized Bed
by Mimi Schwartz

*My Ruby Slippers: Finding Place
on the Road Back to Kansas*
by Tracy Seeley

The Fortune Teller's Kiss
by Brenda Serotte

*Gang of One: Memoirs of
a Red Guard*
by Fan Shen

Just Breathe Normally
by Peggy Shumaker

Scraping By in the Big Eighties
by Natalia Rachel Singer

In the Shadow of Memory
by Floyd Skloot

*Secret Frequencies:
A New York Education*
by John Skoyles

The Days Are Gods
by Liz Stephens

Phantom Limb
by Janet Sternburg

*Yellowstone Autumn: A Season of
Discovery in a Wondrous Land*
by W. D. Wetherell

To order or obtain more information on these or other
University of Nebraska Press titles, visit nebraskapress.unl.edu.

OTHER WORKS BY SONYA HUBER

Opa Nobody

*Cover Me: A Health
Insurance Memoir*

*The Backwards Research Guide
for Writers: Using Your Life for
Reflection, Connection,
and Inspiration*

*Two Eyes Are Never Enough:
A Minimum-Wage Memoir*

*The Evolution of
Hillary Rodham Clinton*

CPSIA information can be obtained
at www.ICGtesting.com
Printed in the USA
LVOW03s1837260318

571193LV00003B/343/P